100 Questions & Answers About Infertility

John D. Gordon, MD

Clinical Professor
Department of Obstetrics and Gynecology
The George Washington University
Co-Director
Dominion Fertility

Michael DiMattina, MD

Clinical Associate Professor
Department of Obstetrics and Gynecology
Georgetown University
Director
Dominion Fertility

JONES AND BARTLETT PUBLISHERS
Sudbury, Massachusetts
BOSTON   TORONTO   LONDON   SINGAPORE

WITHDRAWN

World Headquarters
Jones and Bartlett Publishers
40 Tall Pine Drive
Sudbury, MA 01776
978-443-5000
info@jbpub.com
www.jbpub.com

Jones and Bartlett Publishers
Canada
6339 Ormindale Way
Mississauga, Ontario L5V 1J2
CANADA

Jones and Bartlett Publishers
International
Barb House, Barb Mews
London W6 7PA
UK

Jones and Bartlett's books and products are available through most bookstores and online booksellers. To contact Jones and Bartlett Publishers directly, call 800-832-0034, fax 978-443-8000, or visit our website, www.jbpub.com.

Substantial discounts on bulk quantities of Jones and Bartlett's publications are available to corporations, professional associations, and other qualified organizations. For details and specific discount information, contact the special sales department at Jones and Bartlett via the above contact information or send an email to specialsales@jbpub.com.

The authors, editor, and publisher have made every effort to provide accurate information. However, they are not responsible for errors, omissions, or for any outcomes related to the use of the contents of this book and take no responsibility for the use of the products and procedures described. Treatments and side effects described in this book may not be applicable to all people; likewise, some people may require a dose or experience a side effect that is not described herein. Drugs and medical devices are discussed that may have limited availability controlled by the Food and Drug Administration (FDA) for use only in a research study or clinical trial. Research, clinical practice, and government regulations often change the accepted standard in this field. When consideration is being given to use of any drug in the clinical setting, the health care provider or reader is responsible for determining FDA status of the drug, reading the package insert, and reviewing prescribing information for the most up-to-date recommendations on dose, precautions, and contraindications, and determining the appropriate usage for the product. This is especially important in the case of drugs that are new or seldom used.

Production Credits
Executive Publisher: Christopher Davis
Associate Editor: Kathy Richardson
Production Director: Amy Rose
Production Assistant: Mike Boblitt
Associate Marketing Manager: Rebecca Wasley
Cover Design: Jon Ayotte
Composition: Appingo

Cover Image: Woman in red © Photodisc,
  Woman in white © Photodisc,
  couple © Yuri Arcurs/Shutterstock, Inc.
Manufacturing Buyer: Therese Connell
Printing and Binding: Malloy, Inc.
Cover Printing: Malloy, Inc.

Library of Congress Cataloging-in-Publication Data
Gordon, John D. (John David)
  100 questions and answers about infertility / John D. Gordon and Michael DiMattina.
    p. cm.
  ISBN-13: 978-0-7637-4304-8
  ISBN-10: 0-7637-4304-6
  1. Infertility—Miscellanea. 2. Human reproduction—Miscellanea. 3. Self-care, Health.
  I. DiMattina, Michael. II. Title. III. Title: One hundred questions and answers about infertility.
  RC899.G6779 2008
  616.6'920076—dc22
                          2007009995
6048
Printed in the United States of America
11 10 09 08 07   10 9 8 7 6 5 4 3 2 1

CONTENTS

Part 1. The Basics   1

Questions 1–7 explain how infertility can affect human reproduction . . .
- How does normal human reproduction work?
- What is infertility?
- How common is infertility?

Part 2: The Fertility Evaluation and Treatment Basics   13

Questions 8–20 describe the tests used to evaluate the infertile couple . . .
- What are typical causes of infertility?
- Which tests are routinely performed on the infertile couple?
- What is ovarian reserve, and how is it tested?

Part 3: Specific Problems: Polycystic Ovarian Syndrome (PCOS)   33

Questions 21–26 explain what PCOS is and how it is evaluated and treated . . .
- What prevents a woman from ovulating normally?
- What is polycystic ovarian syndrome?
- Where does PCOS come from, and how is it treated?

Part 4: Specific Problems: Tubal Disease   43

Questions 27–30 describe what can be done in cases of blocked or damaged fallopian tubes . . .
- Can fallopian tubes be repaired?
- Why should blocked fallopian tubes be repaired before IVF is attempted?
- If I had my tubes tied, can I have them untied?

About two weeks ago, a patient asked me to recommend a book that would answer all her basic questions about infertility. She wanted one that was up-to-date, comprehensive, and truly honest about the success rates of the various treatments; but most importantly, she wanted a book to guide her through her journey and to help her make the decisions she needed to make. She wanted the facts, presented in an understandable and logical fashion.

While she was sitting in my office, I went online and searched for that book, the one that would meet her needs. There were a variety of books on infertility, lots of books in fact, but none of them was "the" book. So I told her about one book that could answer some of her questions, another book to answer other questions, etc. But neither of us was particularly satisfied with this plan.

And as so often happens in my life, a few hours later I received a phone call asking if I would be willing to review a new book, a book that aimed to accurately answer the most common questions about infertility. It is obvious that I said yes, because the book you are holding is that book.

I read this book cover to cover (and in such detail that I have to admit I actually asked the authors to tweak it here and there to cover things like mind/body to my satisfaction!) because I feel incredibly strongly that those who are experiencing infertility deserve to be well educated. The reproductive system is so complicated that one of the infertility physicians I work with often remarks that it is a miracle any of us were conceived naturally! You don't need to have an advanced degree to understand it, but if you are undergoing an infertility workup or treatment, you need to know enough to feel comfortable with the plan.

Many of my patients get the vast majority of their information from the Internet, which is fine if that information is accurate. Unfortunately, that is often not the case. Some research has shown that more than 50% of the medical information found online is not correct. Occasionally I lurk on some of the more popular chat rooms, and I have been disturbed to see some of the myths and exaggerations repeated over and over. It would be so nice if indeed a certain herb could treat high follicle-stimulating hormone (FSH) levels and lead to viable pregnancies; it would be terrific if clomiphene would always work if you just give it enough time or increase the dose enough.

Fortunately, if you receive treatment from a physician appropriately trained in infertility treatment, you have an excellent chance of becoming a parent. Unfortunately, that physician often doesn't have the time to answer every single one of your questions.

The goal of *100 Questions and Answers About Infertility* is to give you the background information you need. If you know the basics about infertility, you can use the time you have with your physician to tailor your questions to *you*: What is *your* diagnosis? What is *your* treatment plan? How does your physician plan to maximize the chances that *you* will successfully conceive?

Use this book as a weapon against your infertility. I wish you the very best of luck.

Alice D. Domar, PhD
Executive Director, Domar Center for
    Complementary Healthcare, Boston IVF
Assistant Professor of Obstetrics, Gynecology, and Reproductive Biology,
    Harvard Medical School
Author, Conquering Infertility

As physicians specializing in Reproductive Endocrinology and Infertility, it has been our privilege to care for thousands of patients during our over 30 combined years of clinical practice. Infertility is an emotionally traumatic life event. Although medical progress in the treatment of infertility has been nothing less than astounding, the toll that infertility can take on a couple's or a woman's emotional, spiritual, psychological, and physical well-being can be extreme. Our patients are always our best teachers. We hope that by sharing with you, the reader of this book, some of the frequent questions that we are asked along with our responses, we can help you navigate the voyage ahead as you pursue the evaluation and treatment of infertility.

Acknowledgments

First of all, we wish to acknowledge the staff at Dominion Fertility and thank them for all of the outstanding work that they do on behalf of our patients. It is easy to look good when you are supported by such caring individuals. Secondly, we wish to extend our heartfelt thanks to Dr. David Adamson and Dr. Alice Domar for their insightful comments about this manuscript and their kind words in the introduction and the foreword, respectively. In addition, we wish to thank Kristin and Carol for their participation in this project and for giving a patient's perspective of fertility treatment. Finally, we would like to thank the staff at Jones and Bartlett Publishing (especially Mike Boblitt, Kathy Richardson, and Chris Davis) for their support and editorial assistance in this project.

John David Gordon, MD
Michael DiMattina, MD

It is a great pleasure to write an introduction to Dr. John Gordon and Dr. Michael DiMattina's book *100 Questions and Answers About Infertility*. I have known these fine physicians for a long time and know of their commitment to the education of patients who are suffering from infertility.

The obvious barriers to most patients facing infertility are physical problems of the ovaries, uterus, and fallopian tubes; other hormonal problems; sperm problems; and/or multiple other, more complex factors. It is essential for physicians to identify the problems causing infertility so that effective, individualized treatments can be recommended to each patient. However, patients cannot give themselves their best chance to conceive a baby unless they understand the proposed treatments and can communicate clearly with their physician.

Every treatment has differences in financial cost, time duration, medical risk, and emotional stress. These factors can be perceived very differently by patients depending on their age, duration of infertility, prior treatments, insurance coverage, causes of infertility, religious or moral values, and emotional commitment to fertility treatment. It is impossible for patients to make appropriate choices unless they have a good understanding of their treatment choices. Knowledge is power, especially for infertility patients.

However, it is very difficult to get good information today. Indeed, while many wonderful advantages have been brought about by the Internet and other sources, we are overwhelmed with inaccurate, incorrect, or even purposely misleading information, often written by self-described "medical experts" or those with a limited personal experience of infertility. The information gained from such sources often provides interesting reading, but is usually of little value—and is potentially harmful—to patients trying to make decisions about their infertility treatment. Harm can come from wasting time, money, or emotional resources on treatments that are not the best choice, may not even be effective, and may be risky.

That is where a book like this one becomes so valuable. Dr. Gordon and Dr. DiMattina have written a book that answers 100 commonly asked questions in a straightforward and easily understandable manner. They have identified these questions based on years of experience with patients. They have developed their answers based on their experience and success, and with an understanding of scientific studies in the literature, evidence-based medicine, and national practice guidelines developed by the American Society for Reproductive Medicine. Furthermore, they have been careful to provide a balanced perspective of the advantages and disadvantages of different treatments. This helps patients understand that often more than one approach may be possible and that their own financial and emotional situations are important considerations in deciding the best treatment for them.

I believe that all infertility patients will benefit from reading this very well-written and comprehensive book. This book answers the questions infertility patients need to know, and this knowledge will help them increase their chances of having a baby. With my sincere wishes for good reading and good luck!

David Adamson, MD, FRCSC, FACOG, FACS
Director, Fertility Physicians of Northern California
Adjunct Clinical Professor, Stanford University
Associate Clinical Professor, University of California at San Francisco

PART ONE

The Basics

How does normal human reproduction work?

What is infertility?

How common is infertility?

More . . .

Ovary

A female reproductive organ that contains eggs and produces reproductive hormones.

Fallopian tube

The conduit that serves as an incubator following release and fertilization of the egg.

Uterus

The pear-shaped organ that contains a growing pregnancy.

Follicles

Fluid-filled structures within the ovary that contain an egg.

Pituitary gland

An organ located at the base of the brain that controls several of the other hormone-producing glands.

1. How does normal human reproduction work?

Norman human female reproduction depends on the correct functioning of four components of a woman's body: the brain, the **ovary**, the **fallopian tube**, and the **uterus**. At the time of her birth, a woman's ovary contains all of the eggs that she will ever have. These eggs are contained within fluid-filled sacs called **follicles**.

Every month, the brain sends out a signal from the **pituitary gland** (a gland located at the base of the brain) stimulating the follicles to grow. Not surprisingly, this hormone is called **follicle-stimulating hormone (FSH)**. Under the influence of FSH, a group of follicles begins to grow, but by the fifth day of the reproductive cycle a single dominant follicle has already been selected. This dominant follicle may be either on the right ovary or the left ovary.

As it grows, the follicle produces an important steroid hormone called **estrogen**. Estrogen causes the lining of the uterus (**endometrium**) to thicken in anticipation of the eventual **implantation** of an embryo.

By mid-cycle, this follicle has grown to a diameter of 20 to 22 mm. At this time the brain releases a second hormone, called **luteinizing hormone (LH)**, from the pituitary gland. LH is the trigger that induces **ovulation**.

Approximately 36 hours after the LH surge, the follicle releases the egg. It is the job of the fallopian tube to trap the egg. If the fallopian tube fails to catch the egg, then pregnancy cannot occur.

The eggs are contained within fluid-filled sacs called follicles.

During intercourse, tens of millions of sperm are deposited in the woman's vagina when her male partner reaches orgasm and ejaculates. While the egg is safely held within the fallopian tube, these sperm swim from the vagina, into the cervix, through the uterus, and up into the fallopian tube, where **fertilization** occurs. (See Figure 1.) Normally, a fertilized egg travels through the fallopian tube for 5 days after fertilization, at which point it reaches the uterus. (A fertilized egg that remains trapped within the fallopian tube is called a tubal pregnancy or **ectopic pregnancy,** and can be a life-threatening condition.) The embryo divides many times along the way. By the time it reaches the uterus, it has grown to hundreds of cells and is called a **blastocyst.**

Once the egg is released from the ovary, the follicle (now called a **corpus luteum**) produces both estrogen and a new hormone: **progesterone.** Progesterone changes the estrogen-primed endometrium, allowing implantation of the embryo and thus permitting pregnancy to occur. If a pregnancy does not arise, then 2 weeks after ovulation, the levels of estrogen and progesterone both fall and a menstrual period ensues, during which the lining of the uterus is shed. Menstrual flow lasts approximately 3 to 5 days in most women.

Overall, human beings are not very fertile, with maximum pregnancy rates of only 20% to 25% per cycle during the years of peak fertility (the second and third decades of life).

Follicle-stimulating hormone (FSH)

A protein hormone that promotes the growth and development of follicles, leading eventually to ovulation.

Estrogen

A steroid hormone produced within the growing follicle that induces growth of the endometrium.

Endometrium

The tissue that lines the uterine cavity and is shed each month with a woman's period.

Implantation

The attachment of the early embryo to the endometrial lining of the uterus.

Luteinizing hormone (LH)

A pituitary hormone that induces ovulation in a mature follicle.

Ovulation

The release of an egg from the follicle.

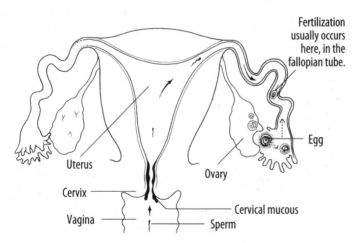

Fertilization usually occurs here, in the fallopian tube.

Egg

Uterus

Ovary

Cervix

Vagina

Cervical mucous

Sperm

**Figure 1   Female Reproductive Organs. Solid arrows indicate path sperm must travel to reach the egg. Dotted arrows indicate path of egg. The fertilized egg continues traveling through the fallopian tube to the uterus.
© 2006 American Society for Reproductive Medicine.**

2. What is infertility?

Approximately 80% to 85% of couples who are trying to become pregnant will successfully conceive within a year. Thus **infertility** is commonly defined as the inability to achieve a pregnancy within 12 months of unprotected intercourse. However, certain patients may have recognized factors that would lead to problems conceiving; for them, the 12-month period of waiting would make no sense. Common examples of such women include those who have extremely irregular periods, a history of severe **endometriosis**, a history of previous tubal pregnancies, or other anatomical factors that would clearly lead to diminished fertility. Couples are encouraged to seek evaluation for infertility if the woman is older than age 35 and they have been attempting pregnancy for a total of 6 months without success.

Another problem related to reproduction is recurrent pregnancy loss. Many women can readily conceive, only to suffer repeated pregnancy losses. These women represent a special subset of those who are unable to successfully reproduce and should be evaluated by a medical professional.

Fertilization

The process by which an egg and a sperm combine and create an embryo.

Ectopic pregnancy

A pregnancy located outside the uterine cavity, usually in the fallopian tube.

Blastocyst

A stage in embryo development reached 5 days after fertilization.

Corpus luteum

The hormone-producing ovarian cyst that forms from the follicle after it releases the egg.

The rate of miscarriage exceeds 50% in women older than age 40.

3. How common is infertility?

Infertility is an extraordinarily common disorder. An estimated 25% of all women will experience an episode of infertility during their lifetime. Infertility currently affects about 6.1 million women and their partners in the United States. The percentage of reproductive-age women who report problems successfully conceiving and delivering a pregnancy varies with age. In the youngest segment of the population, approximately 10% to 15% are affected by this problem. Among women older than age 35, however, more than one-third report diminished fertility. The rates of pregnancy loss are also related to a woman's age, with the rate of miscarriage exceeding 50% in women older than age 40.

Kristin comments:

When you're in the throes of infertility, desperately wanting a child while seemingly everybody around you gets pregnant on their "first try," you wonder if you're the only one who can't get pregnant. My husband and I have been very open about our fertility problems, and once I really started to share our story with friends and acquaintances I discovered I was not alone . . . far from it. I have created amazing friendships with other "infertiles" I have met through Internet communities, reading blogs, and even support groups in my area.

4. Is infertility becoming more common?

A common misperception is that infertility is becoming more common. In fact, the infertility rate has held relatively stable over the years. Instead, two major factors account for the increased utilization of fertility services.

The first of these factors is simply the greater availability of the services themselves. Prior to the 1978 birth of Louise Brown, the world's first baby conceived through **in vitro fertilization (IVF)**, the options available to treat the infertile couple were limited to tubal microsurgery and **ovulation induction** with medications such as clomiphene citrate (Clomid). With the development of **advanced reproductive technologies (ART)**, the techniques used to treat the infertile couple have become both much more successful and more accessible. Fertility providers now practice throughout nearly all urban centers in the continental United States, with more than 400 IVF clinics reporting their success rates through the Society for Assisted Reproductive Technologies (SART) and the Centers for Disease Control and Prevention (CDC). Statistics are available at http://www.cdc.gov/ART/index.htm.

The second factor accounting for the increased use of fertility services is the trend toward delayed childbearing. Over the last generation, a significant number of women have deferred

Progesterone
A steroid hormone produced by the ovary necessary for successful embryo implantation.

Infertility
The inability of a couple to conceive after 12 months of unprotected intercourse.

Endometriosis
The presence of endometrial tissue outside of the endometrial cavity.

In vitro fertilization (IVF)
A fertility treatment in which an egg is placed with a sperm cell in a laboratory culture dish, cultured for several days, and subsequently placed into the uterus.

Ovulation induction
The use of fertility medications to restore normal ovulation in a woman who does not have regular cycles.

Advanced reproductive technologies (ART)
Fertility procedures (including IVF) that involve manipulating sperm and eggs to achieve pregnancy.

childbearing while they pursued advanced academic careers or entered the workplace. Unfortunately, female reproductive capacity drops from a peak in the second and third decades of life so that by the age of 40 years there is a marked reduction in fertility and an increased risk of miscarriage.

The stigma associated with fertility treatments themselves has also eased in recent years, prompting more couples to seek out such help. Previously, couples who were seeking fertility treatments often found themselves beset by a bewildering array of options and knew few other couples with whom they could discuss the range of treatments. Today, more than 100,000 cycles of ART are performed in the United States every year. Given that 1% of all U.S. births are now the result of fertility treatments, most couples probably know someone with a successful outcome from fertility treatments. The current explosion of information available through the Internet and through organizations such as the American Society for Reproductive Medicine (ASRM), RESOLVE, and the American Fertility Association has allowed patients to better understand fertility-related problems and seek appropriate care. A number of states have implemented mandates that guarantee varying levels of insurance coverage for fertility-related procedures, which has had the effect of easing the financial burden for couple who seek out this type of care.

More than 100,000 cycles of ART are performed in the United States every year.

Kristin comments:

When I started discussing my fertility problems with my mother, she opened up about her own struggles to conceive my brother and me. While she did eventually get pregnant on her own, it took her over 2 years to conceive me and about the same amount of time to conceive my brother. She said that nobody really talked about infertility when she was trying to get pregnant and the fertility options were minimal. My mother was an only child because my grandmother could never become pregnant again despite years of trying. I would guess that both my grandmother and my mother had the same infertility diagnosis as I do—PCOS [polycystic ovarian syndrome]—but in their childbearing years it was not commonly diagnosed and treatments were either nonexistent or limited.

5. Who should evaluate the infertile couple?

In many cases, the routine fertility evaluation can be conducted by an obstetrician/gynecologist, a family practitioner, or a **reproductive endocrinologist** (RE). Certain tests can easily be obtained by physicians in the first two specialties, but a reproductive endocrinologist may be required to interpret advanced testing and provide the most accurate counseling. Women who are more than 34 years old may elect to immediately consult with a reproductive endocrinologist.

Reproductive endocrinologist

A physician who specializes in disorders of reproduction, including infertility.

Carol comments:

I began discussions with my gynecologist at age 34 regarding my lack of success at getting pregnant. He put me on a plan that seemed to represent a pretty standard process of elimination. First, I did the basal body temperature charting for 3 months to determine if I was ovulating; then, I spent 3 months on Clomid with no success. Looking back on it now, I question his resistance to send me directly to an RE for further evaluation given my age and what the ovulation charting had revealed. Don't be afraid to push your doctors. I wish I would have pushed harder to get things moving.

6. What is a reproductive endocrinologist?

A reproductive endocrinologist (RE) is a physician who specializes in the treatment of reproductive disorders and infertility. To specialize as a reproductive endocrinologist, a physician undergoes 4 years of training in general obstetrics and gynecology following his or her completion of medical school. At the end of these 4 years of training (internship and residency), which includes exposure to normal and high-risk obstetrics, gynecology, gynecologic oncology, and reproductive endocrinology and infertility, a physician must then apply for an additional 3-year fellowship in reproductive endocrinology and infertility. After completing these 7 years of training, the physician takes a series of written and oral examinations to become board certified in this specialty. Although not all practitioners of reproductive endocrinology and infertility have undergone formal fellowship-level training, the majority have, and this training includes both clinical and basic science experience.

There are several professional organizations for physicians who are interested in the treatment of the infertile couple, including the American Society of Reproductive Medicine (ASRM) and the Society for Reproductive Endocrinology and Infertility (SREI). Any physician who is interested in infertility may join ASRM, but members of SREI must be board eligible or board certified in reproductive endocrinology and infertility. Both of these organizations maintain websites that allow patients to identify local specialists (www.asrm.org; www.socrei.org).

Members of SREI must be board eligible or board certified in reproductive endocrinology and infertility.

7. How do I choose a fertility clinic?

Choosing a fertility doctor for your care may be the single most important factor that leads to a successful pregnancy, so choose carefully.

Many patients are referred to us by their OB/GYN, friends, relatives, former patients, news articles, or through the Internet. But the one common denominator we have routinely observed with the sophisticated patient is that she is well prepared before coming for her initial office visit or she quickly becomes informed and knowledgeable before we begin any treatments. Patients often say to us, "I checked you out before making this appointment." Of course, we are always flattered by such comments, but we know that this patient will ask all of the important questions and make an intelligent decision regarding her treatment options. She will also probably experience less stress during the evaluation and treatment process, as she has developed a better knowledge base and understanding of what to expect.

All fertility clinics come with a unique flavor of their own. Some are run by a solo practitioner, others by 2 to 6 member groups, while others are clinics with over 15 doctors. Regardless of the size of the group, be sure you are getting the attention and treatments you desire and deserve. You should never feel like a number with a revolving door of doctors.

Of course, patients are not doctors and will not have the knowledge or experience of a reproductive endocrinologist, but a caring doctor will always welcome any and all questions and will take the time to answer them in a way that you can understand. We view patients as our partners, and once we understand what they are willing or not willing to do, we can devise a treatment plan that offers hope without subjecting them to any unnecessary additional stress.

A caring doctor will always welcome any and all questions and will take the time to answer them in a way that you can understand.

Other things to consider.

Statistics, statistics, statistics: You want a baby, so choose a fertility clinic with good success rates. However, a wise man once said: "There are lies, damn lies, and statistics." So, how does one determine what to make of these statistics? In truth, there is no easy answer. Clinics that are more selective can inflate their success rates, while those that have a different philosophy may suffer the consequences even though they have an excellent program. When considering a clinic, it is important to know what your specific chances for success will be within that clinic.

If there is one yardstick to compare clinics, then that is the pregnancy rate using donor eggs. In this patient population, the pregnancy rates should be very high. A low donor egg pregnancy rate may be concerning.

Advertising may be misleading. Obviously, a practice with 10 to 20 doctors will produce more total babies than a medical practice with only 2 to 6 fertility doctors, but the pregnancy rates may be equivalent (as can be seen in Figure 37 of Appendix B). Individuals should evaluate the clinic statistics and obtain a good understanding and feel for what their specific chances for pregnancy will be per treatment. Patients may also evaluate the clinic success by reviewing IVF statistics at the Centers for Disease Control and Prevention (www.cdc. gov/ART/index.htm/).

Experience: Experience of the clinic, in our opinion, may be one of the most important factors when deciding which doctor and which clinic to seek for fertility care. One should ask how long the doctors have been performing various treatment procedures. It is also important to know whether or not cutting edge procedures are either being offered or are being developed in the practice.

Subspecialty board certification: Most doctors practicing in the field of in vitro fertilization and infertility are subspecialty board certified in reproductive endocrinology and infertility. This certification can be found by going to the Society for Reproductive Endocrinology's Web site, which lists doctors who are subspecialty certified in reproductive endocrinology and infertility. Additionally, patients may find it beneficial to check if their doctor has a faculty position at one of the local medical universities or actively participates in the teaching of the medical students and residents in their locality.

It is important that you have access to your doctor.

Availability and accessibility of doctors: It is important that you have access to your doctor in order to have your questions answered and needs addressed. Evaluate whether or not the availability and accessibility of the doctor is an easy process or a difficult one when making decisions as to where to seek care. The friendliness and helpfulness of the staff will also give you a feel for the character of the practice.

Intracytoplasmic sperm injection (ICSI)

The injection of a sperm into an egg, in IVF cases when fertilization might not otherwise occur.

Cost: It is always important to get the *total* cost. Factor in extra expenses such as the fertility drugs, which can cost thousands of dollars; intracytoplasmic sperm injection (ICSI); assisted embryo hatching; embryo cryopreservation; and preimplantation genetic diagnosis (PDD). These drugs and procedures can quickly increase the overall cost for treatment.

A word of caution: In general, Internet chat rooms may be a dangerous place for seeking advice regarding finding an infertility doctor. Be careful what you hear online, as it always represents just one half of the story. It is far better for you to do your own homework and research than to rely on information provided from others, which may be based on misleading impressions or experiences.

PART TWO

The Fertility Evaluation and Treatment Basics

What are typical causes of infertility?

Which tests are routinely performed
on the infertile couple?

What is ovarian reserve, and how is it tested?

More . . .

8. What are typical causes of infertility?

The causes of infertility are wide ranging but can be examined in light of the reproductive cycle described in Question 1. (See Table 1.) In general, the causes of infertility can be equally divided between the male and female partners in a couple.

Table 1   Etiology: Infertility Diagnosis Reported Among Couples Who Had an ART Procedure Using Non-donor Eggs or Embryos in 2004.

Cause of Infertility	%
Female factors (single)	32
• Tubal factor	11
• Endometriosis	6
• Ovulatory dysfunction	6
• Diminished ovarian reserve	8
• Uterine factor	1
Male factor (single)	19
Other cause(s)[a]	7
Unexplained cause[b]	12
Multiple factors (female only)	12
Multiple factors (female + male)	18

[a]Includes immunologic problems, chromosomal abnormalities, cancer chemotherapy, and serious illness.
[b]No cause of infertility found in either partner.
Source: Adapted from the Centers for Disease Control and Prevention. 2004 Assisted Reproductive Technology Success Rates, December 2006.

The causes of infertility can be equally divided between the male and female partners in a couple.

Half of all infertility cases, therefore, involve problems with the sperm of the male partner. Unfortunately, functional tests for sperm competence (the ability of sperm to fertilize an egg) are not available. Thus, when assessing male-related fertility issues, a semen analysis determines the total number of sperm (concentration), the percentage of those sperm that are moving (motility), and the shape of the sperm (morphology).

Many factors can reduce the female partner's ability to conceive. For example, a woman may have anatomical problems related to the fallopian tubes, uterus, and peritoneal structures within the pelvis such as **adhesions** or endometriosis. Problems with ovulation are very common in infertile patients, and women with irregular periods may suffer from a common disorder such as **polycystic ovarian syndrome (PCOS)**. Another factor often found in conjunction with infertility is reproductive aging. A woman's peak years of fertility occur when she is in her twenties. A woman's fertility declines significantly during her thirties and forties, with an especially rapid decline in fertility occurring after she passes age 35.

9. Which tests are routinely performed on the infertile couple?

The basic infertility evaluation consists of a handful of tests: **transvaginal ultrasound**, blood tests, an assessment of the fallopian tubes (for the female partner), and **semen analysis** (for the male partner).

Transvaginal ultrasound allows the physician to assess the appearance of the uterus and the ovaries. During this examination, the physician may discover uterine abnormalities such as **fibroids** (benign growths of the muscle of the uterus) or uterine polyps (benign growths of the lining of the uterus). **Ultrasonography** can also identify the location of the ovaries and determine the number of follicles present (**antral follicle count**), which correlates with the woman's response to fertility medications. In addition, examination of the ovaries may reveal the presence of abnormal ovarian cysts such as **endometriomas**, dermoid cysts, or—in rare cases—precancerous and cancerous lesions.

In addition to the routine vaginal ultrasound, an assessment of the fallopian tubes and the uterus cavity is appropriate when the woman is having trouble conceiving. This examination is usually accomplished through a **hysterosalpingogram** (HSG: see Figure 2), an x-ray test that is performed under fluoroscopy by either the fertility physician or a radiologist. Although it may sometimes cause mild uterine cramping, the vast majority of patients tolerate this procedure without difficulty.

Adhesions

Bands of fibrous tissue that can bind reproductive organs, thereby reducing a woman's fertility.

Polycystic ovarian syndrome (PCOS)

A common gynecologic disorder often leading to irregular periods and infertility.

Transvaginal ultrasound

An imaging technique that uses sound waves produced by a wand-like probe placed within the vagina.

Semen analysis

A laboratory test used to assess male fertility. It usually includes evaluation of the sperm volume, pH, concentration, motility and morphology in a sample.

Fibroids

Benign growths of the connective tissue of the uterus.

Ultrasonography

A noninvasive imaging technology that uses sound waves to create images of various structures in the body.

Alternatives to the hysterosalpingogram include **laparoscopy** and **hysteroscopy**; these outpatient surgical procedures are described in Questions 10 and 11.

Laboratory tests on the female partner of an infertile couple usually include routine screening tests such as those for blood type, blood count, and rubella immunity. In addition, most physicians perform tests that check the woman's **prolactin** and **thyroid-stimulating hormone (TSH)** levels. Additional reproductive hormone testing for **ovarian reserve** is usually part of the routine evaluation as well (see Question 9).

Routine testing of the male partner of an infertile couple includes a basic semen analysis evaluating the volume of semen, the concentration of sperm (sperm count), the percentage of moving sperm (**sperm motility**), and the percentage of normally shaped sperm (**sperm morphology**). (See Table 2.) Although some clinics perform additional sperm function tests, such as the **acrosome reaction** and **hypo-osmotic swelling test**, the overall benefit of these two tests remains somewhat controversial. Both of these tests attempt to predict the functional ability of the sperm in terms of its ability to fertilize an egg. Ultimately, however, the best evidence of normal sperm function is a recent pregnancy or normal fertilization during a cycle of IVF.

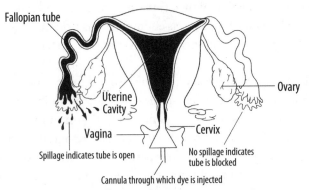

Figure 2   HSG, a procedure to determine if the fallopian tubes are open or blocked. © 2006 American Society for Reproductive Medicine.

Table 2 Components of the Routine Semen Analysis

Parameter	Reference Value
Volume	1.5–5.0 mL (pH, 7.2)
Concentration	> 20 million/mL
Total motile count	10 million
Motility	> 50%
Normal morphology	> 30% normal (World Health Organization, 1999)
	> 14% normal (Kruger and Coetzee, 1999)
Indirect immuno-bead assay (sperm antibodies	≥ 20%

Source: Adapted from World Health Organization. *WHO Laboratory Manual for the Examination of Human Semen and Semen-Cervical Mucus Interaction.* New York: Cambridge University Press, 1999.

Tests to detect the presence of **antisperm antibodies** in the blood of the female partner or coating the individual sperm may sometimes be recommended. Female antisperm antibodies may cause infertility that is best treated by IVF. Antisperm antibodies present on the sperm themselves may inhibit normal fertilization. In such cases, collecting a semen sample in media for use in **artificial insemination** may be considered, but most of these patients pursue IVF with intracytoplasmic sperm injection (ICSI).

Kristin comments:

Despite having a diagnosis of PCOS when I was referred to an RE, I still had to go through the regular battery of blood tests, ultrasounds, and an HSG. It was a really scary time because none of my friends had ever gone through any of the tests and I really felt like a pincushion. Besides the physical toll of the tests, it was definitely emotionally draining. I think the initial tests in some ways prepare you for the weeks of daily blood draws and ultrasounds that accompany IUI [intra-uterine insemination] and IVF. Before IVF I was terrified of needles, but within days I was a pro at giving myself shots.

Thyroid-stimulating hormone (TSH)

A hormone produced by the pituitary gland that stimulates the production of thyroid hormone from the thyroid gland.

Ovarian reserve

The fertility potential of a woman as determined by both the number of her ovarian follicles and the health of the eggs located within those follicles.

Sperm motility

The movement of sperm when viewed under a microscope.

The best evidence of normal sperm function is a recent pregnancy or normal fertilization during a cycle of IVF.

Sperm morphology

The shape and outward appearance of the sperm when viewed under a microscope.

10. What is ovarian reserve, and how is it tested?

During a woman's reproductive cycle, each month a single follicle is selected out of a group of potential follicles, reaches maturity, and ovulates a single egg. Many fertility treatments use medications to "rescue" other follicles from that group, so that multiple eggs are released during ovulation as opposed to just a single egg. If physicians could predict which patients would respond well to fertility treatments, then those women with a poor chance of success could defer these treatments and consider other options. Those women who respond well to fertility medications are described as having normal ovarian reserve. Those patients who have a poor response to fertility medications are described as having **diminished ovarian reserve**.

Ovarian reserve consists of two separate components, both of which determine a woman's chance of conceiving a child with IVF. The first component is the number of extra follicles that are available to undergo recruitment with treatment using fertility medications. This number depends on several factors, including the woman's chronological age (as discussed below), previous ovarian surgery, genetics, and exposure to environmental toxins (most notably, tobacco usage).

The second component is the actual health of the follicles and the eggs within those follicles. First and foremost, egg quality is determined by a woman's chronological age. Peak female fertility occurs when a woman is in her twenties and then drops significantly with age, especially following age 35. This fact has been conclusively demonstrated in many ways but is especially obvious when we look at IVF pregnancy rates. In patients who undergo IVF, studies have shown that around the age of 35 years old a marked decrease occurs in the chance of an embryo implanting successfully. In addition, the miscarriage rate rises with age, especially in those women older than age 40, in whom this rate exceeds 50%. Therefore, the age component of ovarian reserve is essentially immutable. In other words, unless she uses eggs from an egg donor, a woman cannot change her chronological age—and with increasing age, the number of normal eggs inevitably falls sharply. Although it is true that the percentage of normal eggs within an ovary is specific to the individual woman, even the most fertile women possess very few normal eggs after age 40.

The concept of ovarian reserve testing, therefore, represents a means by which the physician attempts to evaluate a woman's reproductive potential both in terms of the number of follicles that remain and the health of those follicles. There are several ways in which one can assess ovarian reserve. First, the woman's follicle-stimulating hormone (FSH) level can be measured on day 2 or 3 of a normal menstrual cycle. An estradiol level should be obtained at the same time, because the FSH level can be misleadingly low in women who have a high estrogen level early in the menstrual cycle. Alternatively, ovarian reserve can be assessed by performing a transvaginal ultrasound and counting the antral follicles present. In women with a slightly elevated FSH level, a transvaginal ultrasound may reveal a large number of follicles—somewhat reassuring the patient and her physician that perhaps her ovarian reserve is more normal than might otherwise be expected.

Unfortunately, normal FSH and estradiol levels do not guarantee a normal response to fertility medications. The **clomiphene citrate challenge test (CCCT)** was initially described as a means to identify those women with normal FSH and estradiol levels on day 3 of the menstrual cycle (**day-3 hormones**) who may demonstrate a suboptimal response to injectable fertility medications and poor IVF pregnancy rates. In the CCCT, the patient takes 100 mg of clomiphene citrate on cycle days 5 through 9. An FSH level is checked on days 3 and 10. If both of these levels are less than 10 IU/L (international units), then this represents a normal response. If the FSH level is greater than 10 IU on day 3 but less than 10 IU on day 10, then this represents a borderline situation, but potentially reassuring based on the response of the ovary

Diminished ovarian reserve

The inability to respond appropriately to fertility medications, both in terms of the number of follicles produced and the health of the eggs.

Clomiphene citrate challenge test (CCCT)

A test used to evaluate a woman's ovarian reserve before she undergoes a fertility treatment.

Day-3 hormones

Measurement of follicle-stimulating hormone and estradiol on the second or third day of a regular menstrual cycle, which provides an assessment of a woman's ovarian reserve.

to stimulation with clomiphene citrate. If the FSH level is normal on day 3 but more than 10 IU on day 10, however, the woman is likely to exhibit a suboptimal response to fertility medication, along with high IVF cancellation rates and poor pregnancy rates.

A word of caution is in order regarding ovarian reserve testing, including the CCCT: Virtually all physicians have patients who have successfully delivered a child following an abnormal CCCT. An abnormal CCCT or elevated FSH levels on cycle day 3 do not preclude spontaneous pregnancy and delivery. Nevertheless, the miscarriage rate and the incidence of Down syndrome may be increased in such pregnancies. Patients with diminished ovarian reserve may have successful treatment with the combination of fertility drugs and intra-uterine insemination (IUI), or even with IUI alone.

The real benefit of the CCCT is its ability to identify those patients in whom IVF is markedly less likely to be successful, allowing them to focus on other options such as donor-egg IVF, adoption, or less invasive office-based fertility treatments. Overall, ovarian reserve testing represents an important factor when considering various fertility treatments and may be the final arbitrator in selecting the specific treatment plan.

The real benefit of the CCCT is its ability to identify those patients in whom IVF is markedly less likely to be successful.

11. What is a laparoscopy, and do I need one?

A laparoscopy is an outpatient surgery usually performed under general anesthesia. Most laparoscopies are completed in a hospital, but some physicians utilize freestanding outpatient surgery centers.

During a laparoscopy, the physician inserts a small fiber-optic telescope into the abdominal cavity through an incision made in the patient's umbilical area (belly button). Most physicians initially distend the abdomen using carbon dioxide gas with a needle (Veres needle) to create what is called a pneumoperitoneum. A trocar—an instrument with a diameter similar to that of a pencil—is then passed through the umbilicus, allowing for introduction of the telescope (called a laparoscope) into the abdomen.

Using the laparoscope, a gynecologic surgeon can inspect the uterus, fallopian tubes, and ovaries. The appendix and upper abdomen are carefully inspected as well. Additional instruments may be inserted into the abdomen through incisions (ports) made along the hairline above the pubic bone. For example, the physician may use graspers, scissors, or suction irrigators to rinse the tissue and remove blood and fluids as needed. Some physicians insert a slightly larger telescope through the umbilical port, which allows them to use a carbon dioxide laser to cut scar tissue or destroy implants of endometriosis. Besides the laser, other instruments can be used to cut or burn abnormalities such as endometriosis or scar tissue.

During a laparoscopy, the physician typically introduces a blue dye into the uterine cavity while directly visualizing the fallopian tubes. If the fallopian tubes are patent (open) but are located in an abnormal location because of scar tissue, then the surgeon may try to free the fallopian tubes to improve the patient's fertility.

If abnormal ovarian cysts such as endometriomas are present, then the physician may remove them during the course of the laparoscopy or, if necessary, perform a **laparotomy**. A laparotomy is a surgery performed through a larger incision, usually made along the bikini line. It may require the patient to stay 1 to 3 days in the hospital following the surgery. In addition, a laparotomy requires a longer recovery period and may create more new scar tissue than laparoscopic surgery.

Certain abnormalities cannot be easily treated through laparoscopy, including exceedingly large ovarian cysts, ovarian cysts that are suspicious for cancer, and fibroids that are deeply embedded in the wall of the uterus. Patients with these problems are probably better served by a laparotomy.

Laparotomy

An inpatient surgical procedure that is performed through an open abdominal incision.

For many years, all women who were seeking fertility care underwent laparoscopy as part of the initial evaluation. In recent times, this practice has faded with increased utilization of IVF. Although IVF has essentially replaced tubal surgery in patients with tubal factor infertility, laparoscopy is still used to correct certain problems in patients prior to undergoing IVF. Complications of laparoscopy are rare but can include injury to the bowel, bladder, and blood vessels; a need for laparotomy; and even death.

12. What is a hysteroscopy, and do I need one? Is it the same as a water sonogram or a hysterosalpingogram?

A hysteroscopy is an outpatient surgical procedure that is performed either to diagnose or to treat a problem within the uterine cavity. During hysteroscopy, the physician inserts a small fiber-optic telescope through the cervix and into the uterus. Either gas or liquid can be used to distend the uterus and allow the physician to directly visualize the uterine cavity. The physician may also introduce small instruments into the uterus to cut scar tissue or remove polyps or fibroids. Although diagnostic hysteroscopy can be performed in the physician's office under local anesthesia, operative hysteroscopy requires anesthesia because of the cramping that occurs during uterine manipulation. Complications of hysteroscopy are rare but may include infection, bleeding, uterine perforation, damage to adjacent structures, and even death.

Hysterosonogram

A type of transvaginal sonogram performed after placement of a small catheter into the uterine cavity through which sterile water is introduced, allowing for visualization of the uterine cavity.

A water sonogram (**hysterosonogram**) is a specialized ultrasound examination performed using a transvaginal ultrasound probe. A small catheter is placed within the uterine cavity, and sterile saline is then introduced into the cavity during the sonogram to allow the physician to visualize any uterine polyps or fibroids. Usually, this kind of examination does not provide any information about the status of the fallopian tubes. Nevertheless, hysterosonograms are helpful in identifying the presence of an endometrialpolyp seen on routine sonogram or the location of a fibroid (see Figure 3). They have limited benefit in evaluating uterine scar tissue and are only diagnostic (not therapeutic).

A hysterosalpingogram (HSG) is similar to a hysterosonogram in that fluid is introduced into the uterine cavity—but that is where the similarity ends. During an HSG, a radioopaque dye is first introduced into the uterus; x-rays are then taken of the area. The HSG can be used to diagnose polyps and fibroids and is superior to hysterosonogram in evaluating the presence of uterine scar tissue. This type of imaging also provides information on the status of the fallopian tubes, unlike either a hysteroscopy or a hysterosonogram. Because it employs traditional x-rays, an HSG is usually performed at a hospital's radiology department or at a radiologist's office, as few REs have this equipment in their offices.

A hysterosalpingogram provides information on the status of the fallopian tubes, unlike either a hysteroscopy or a hysterosonogram.

13. What is ureaplasma, and how did I get it?

Most reproductive endocrinologists routinely obtain samples from the cervix (cervical cultures) to assess their patients for **gonorrhea, chlamydia, ureaplasma, mycoplasma,** and other bacteria. Gonorrhea and chlamydia are sexually transmitted diseases that can cause tubal damage and infertility when these infections are passed back and forth between sexually intimate partners. Patients with gonorrhea may have a yellowish discharge associated with pelvic pain and fever. Although chlamydia can be associated with these symptoms,

Gonorrhea

A sexually transmitted disease that can cause tubal damage and infertility.

Chlamydia

A common sexually transmitted disease that can damage a woman's fallopian tubes.

Ureaplasma

A type of bacteria that may contribute to infertility.

Mycoplasma

A type of bacteria that may contribute to infertility.

Figure 3   Sonohysterography showing a fibroid extending into the uterine cavity. © 2006 American Society for Reproductive Medicine.

chlamydial infections are often silent; despite their lack of symptoms, these infections may result in significant tubal scarring and damage.

Ureaplasma and mycoplasma are somewhat more problematic to label as reproductive tract pathogens, because they are often found in fertile, healthy couples in addition to those with infertility. These bacteria have been hypothesized to play a role in both infertility and miscarriage, but the specific mechanisms by which they alter fertility are unclear. Whether ureaplasma or mycoplasma can cause reproductive tract damage or whether their presence increases the rate of miscarriage is controversial. As a consequence, many clinics do not test for ureaplasma or mycoplasma routinely.

If the cultures for ureaplasma and mycoplasma are positive, both the patient and her sexual partner are treated with antibiotics. As these bacteria may have been present for many years without causing any symptoms, the finding of ureaplasma and mycoplasma on cervical cultures does not in any way indicate infidelity or sexual misconduct.

14. Can infertility be unexplained?

Although the etiology (underlying source) of infertility in many couples can be elucidated by various forms of testing, including careful physical examination and history, there still remains a sizable percentage of couples in whom no obvious cause of infertility can be identified. Some studies estimate that approximately 10% to 20% of patients fall into this category. However, "unexplained infertility" is not necessarily equivalent to "untreatable infertility." If a couple has prolonged, unexplained infertility with no previous pregnancies, then a number of etiologies are possible.

Approximately 10% to 20% of couples have unexplained infertility.

If the woman is having normal, regular menstrual cycles, it is likely that an egg is growing and being released in an appropriate fashion. If pregnancy has never occurred, however, we cannot be sure that the woman's fallopian tubes are able to catch the egg or that her male partner's sperm are able to swim through the cervix and uterus and find the egg in the fallopian tube (where fertilization normally occurs). If the sperm is able to reach the egg, the absence of a previous pregnancy raises the question as to whether fertilization can, in fact, occur. The scope of this problem is made clear when we look at the fertilization results for patients who undergo IVF. Typically the rate of failed fertilization with IVF is approximately 2%, but this rate increases dramatically—to approximately 20%—in couples who have prolonged infertility with no previous pregnancies. Failed fertilization can be the result of a problem with either the sperm or the egg, or both. Since the introduction of intracytoplasmic sperm injection (ICSI; described later in this book), however, the specific causes of fertilization failure are not as important as the fact that we have a means to avoid this unfortunate outcome in most cases.

One of the most significant developments in the treatment of infertile couples has been the move away from extensive diagnostic testing and toward a more rapid recommendation to undergo IVF. We often recommend that patients with prolonged unexplained infertility consider IVF with ICSI, as this combination has both diagnostic and therapeutic benefits.

Carol comments:

We were never able to diagnose the exact reason that I couldn't become pregnant. This can be frustrating and scary because there is no clear-cut path to fixing a problem that you can't define. I remember talking to other women who had more defined issues such as male factor or PCOS and thinking that those would be easier diagnoses to deal with. Luckily, we were able to benefit from the movement to more rapidly recommend undergoing IVF for patients whose infertility is unexplained.

The combination of in vitro fertilization and intracytoplasmic sperm injection may have both diagnostic and therapeutic benefits.

15. After we have sex, I think that everything comes out. Can this prevent pregnancy?

At the time of orgasm, the human male's ejaculation is composed of proteins, enzymes, and water from the seminal vesicles. The sperm represent only one to three drops of the total ejaculate volume of 1.5 to 5 mL. The sperm immediately move from the vagina and enter the cervical mucus, where they can live for 5 to 7 days. The cervical mucus serves as a reservoir for the sperm, from which they can subsequently ascend to the upper reproductive tract and meet the egg in the fallopian tube.

It is normal for much of the ejaculate to spill out of the vagina following coitus. For most couples, this does not decrease their chances for pregnancy. Rarely, a woman may have a prolapsed vagina that cannot support and hold enough of the ejaculate following coitus. Such conditions usually occur only after several previous vaginal deliveries.

16. My friend keeps asking whether I had an endometrial biopsy or a postcoital test. Do I need these tests?

Endometrial biopsy

A sample of the lining of the uterus, usually performed to rule out endometrial cancer.

Postcoital test

A test of historical interest used to assess the presence and behavior of sperm found within the cervical mucus.

Many couples ask their physicians about performing an **endometrial biopsy** or a **postcoital test**. Unfortunately, both of these tests have limited benefit in assessing the infertile couple.

An endometrial biopsy is performed just before the onset of a woman's menses and represents an attempt to identify an abnormality of the lining of her uterus. The problem with the endometrial biopsy in terms of its usefulness as a fertility test is that abnormal biopsies are obtained in more than one-third of women with proven fertility. Therefore, the finding of an abnormal endometrial biopsy in fertility patients is of uncertain benefit. Most reproductive endocrinologists prefer to have their patients take extra progesterone, essentially obviating the need for the endometrial biopsy. At the present time, this test is most useful as a means to rule out endometrial cancer in those patients who are at increased risk of this disease. Patients at increased risk for endometrial cancer include those who have polycystic ovarian syndrome and infrequent, heavy periods but who do not receive the protective benefit of oral contraceptives or other progesterone-containing medications.

The postcoital test was initially proposed as a means to evaluate the interaction of the male partner's sperm and the female partner's cervical mucus. This test is performed approximately 8 to 24 hours after intercourse at midcycle (around days 12 to 14 of the menstrual cycle). During a speculum exam, the physician collects a sample of cervical mucus. This sample is then placed on a slide and examined under a microscope for the presence of motile sperm. In addition to the presence or absence of sperm, the physician records the quality, quantity, and appearance of the mucus. Unfortunately, the postcoital test has very poor reproducibility and limited utility in the evaluation of infertile couples. Couples for whom no motile sperm were observed during the postcoital test have conceived, for example. Although the spontaneous pregnancy rates are higher in those patients with a normal postcoital test, the information gathered in this way seldom provides any useful insight when developing a therapeutic plan.

The postcoital test has very poor reproducibility and limited utility in the evaluation of infertile couples.

Postcoital tests may prove more valuable in couples in whom, for social or religious reasons, the male partner is unable to provide a specimen for semen analysis. In these cases, a postcoital test reassures all parties that sperm are actually deposited in the vagina during the act of intercourse.

17. Can I choose the sex of my baby?

Gender is determined at the moment of fertilization, when a sperm bearing either an X or Y **chromosome** penetrates the egg, resulting in formation of either a female or male embryo, respectively. The event is random, and the sex ratio of females to males conceived is fairly even.

Chromosomes
One of the threadlike "packages" of genes and other DNA in the nucleus of a cell. Humans have 23 pairs of chromosomes, for a total of 46 in all: 44 autosomes and 2 sex chromosomes.

Several techniques exist that can enhance the likelihood that a couple will conceive a child with the desired gender. The Ericsson method is a simple, noninvasive method that separates X-bearing sperm from Y-bearing sperm using centrifugation techniques. The sperm are placed on the top of a column of either albumin or Sephadex, and the specimen is centrifuged to isolate the desired gender-selected sperm. These sperm are then placed in the female partner through intrauterine insemination. The success rates reported with this method vary from no benefit to as high as 75% for the desired gender. The Ericsson method is not associated with any known risk to either baby or mother.

A newer experimental technique (Microsort) involves the labeling of the DNA of the sperm, followed by passage of the sample through a cell-sorting machine. This process yields a smaller sperm sample than the Ericsson method, and IVF with ICSI may be required for pregnancy. Nevertheless, the results appear encouraging in terms of gender selection.

Preimplantation genetic diagnosis (PGD)

Evaluation of the genetic status of an embryo prior to its implantation, usually through the removal of 1 to 2 cells at the 8-cell stage of development. The isolated cells can then be analyzed for specific chromosomal conditions and other genetic disorders.

The gender of a child can also be selected using IVF and **preimplantation genetic diagnosis (PGD)**. This technique is expensive and much more complex than the Ericsson method, but success rates for the selected gender routinely exceed 90%. Couples who elect to pursue IVF and PGD for gender selection often do so to prevent genetically inheritable medical diseases, such as Duchenne muscular dystrophy, from occurring in their children.

Many medical authorities consider gender selection to be unethical except in a few circumstances, such as when the couple runs a high risk of having a child with an inheritable medical disease. Others support the use of gender selection when a couple has at least one child but want to limit their family size and desire a child of the opposite gender.

18. How will my reproductive endocrinologist determine a plan of therapy?

In general, reproductive endocrinologists recommend a particular course of treatment only after obtaining the results from the full spectrum of fertility tests. In general, these tests include a pelvic ultrasound, an assessment of tubal patency (hysterosalpingogram or laparoscopy), a semen analysis, and a variety of blood tests.

The therapeutic plan for any couple is unique to them. If testing has demonstrated a clear problem, such as blocked fallopian tubes or a markedly abnormal sperm count, then in vitro fertilization (IVF) may be recommended as the only reasonable alternative. However, most couples are not sterile but merely subfertile, so they may be offered a range of therapeutic options—from expectant management, to the use of insemination with or without fertility drugs, to IVF with or without intracytoplasmic sperm injection (ICSI). IVF can be performed using the patient's own eggs, donor eggs, or donor sperm.

Most couples are not sterile but merely subfertile, so they may be offered a range of therapeutic options.

A couple's particular therapeutic plan will be developed with their specific needs in mind. For those patients in whom IVF is not an option, whether because of religious, financial, or philosophical reasons, the physician will offer counseling about the alternative treatments available to them. Not all couples are prepared to undergo extensive treatments for their infertility, so their physician will likely tailor the options appropriately when proposing a course of action to a particular couple. Given that infertile couples can sometimes achieve spontaneous pregnancies, the desire of a couple to proceed with therapy needs to be weighed against the likelihood of success for that therapy and the cost involved. These costs may include financial, physical, and emotional considerations.

Carol comments:

I feel that finding an RE who will work with you and listen to you is one of the most important factors in achieving a positive outcome. Each individual who is faced with infertility deals with the varying costs (financial, physical, and emotional) differently. For some, the financial aspect limits the number or attempts they can make. For others, the physical and emotional aspects take such a toll that they are only willing to go through a set number of attempts. Based on my discussions with other women who have faced fertility challenges, I believe that each person has a unique threshold for these costs. If you are dealing with a doctor who strictly adheres to a "one size fits all" policy and won't take your personal situation into consideration, it will only add more stress to an already stressful situation.

19. How expensive are infertility treatments?

Some insurance plans may cover the cost of fertility treatments. In those patients without insurance coverage, the cost of fertility treatments varies widely depending on the specific treatment utilized. For example, a cycle of ultrasound monitoring without the use of fertility medications, culminating with **intrauterine insemination (IUI)**, may cost $1300 to $1500 in many clinics. Compare this with the cost of IVF with intracytoplasmic sperm injection, freezing of extra embryos, and assisted embryo hatching, for which the price tag can total $14,000 to $16,000, which must then be added to the cost of injectable fertility medications ($2000 to $4000). The use of **donor-egg IVF**, although extremely successful, is also very expensive, because the donor must be reimbursed for her time and effort as part of the treatment and also because of the extreme screening tests mandated by the FDA. The price for donor-egg IVF typically ranges between $25,000 and $30,000, depending on the clinic.

In most cases, the more expensive, more invasive fertility treatments usually result in the highest pregnancy rates. Couples are advised to carefully consider the proposed course of treatment and the costs that may be involved.

Many IVF centers in the United States offer "money back" (refund) programs. A couple accepted into such a program pays a premium that covers several fresh IVF cycles as well as **frozen embryo transfers (FET)**. If they fail to conceive or are deemed to no longer be appropriate candidates for

Intrauterine insemination (IUI)

A fertility treatment in which the sperm are washed and then placed within the uterine cavity.

Donor-egg IVF

An extremely successful type of in vitro fertilization procedure using the eggs from a young woman and with the resulting embryo(s) transferred into the recipient.

Some insurance plans may cover the cost of fertility treatments.

Frozen embryo transfer (FET)

Placement of previously cryopreserved embryos into the uterus or, more rarely, the fallopian tube.

treatment, then all or a percentage of their initial payment is refunded. These programs have remained somewhat controversial but can allow couples to pursue other options if IVF proves unsuccessful.

According to the ASRM Ethics Committee Statement of June 2006, the controversy surrounding such programs relates in part to the concern that such arrangements appear to violate long-standing ethical prohibitions against paying contingency fees in medicine. This concern is based on Opinion 6.01 of the AMA Code of Medical Ethics, which states, "a physician's fee should not be made contingent on the successful outcome of a medical treatment."

Furthermore, the Committee Statement (which can be found on the ASRM website at http://www.asrm.org/Media/Ethics/ethicsmain.html) concludes, "the risk-sharing form of payment for IVF is an option that might be ethically offered to patients without health insurance coverage for IVF if certain conditions that protect patient interests are met. These conditions are that the criterion of success is clearly specified, that patients are fully informed of the financial costs and advantages and disadvantages of such programs, that informed consent materials clearly inform patients of their chances of success if found eligible for the risk-sharing program, and that the program is not guaranteeing pregnancy and delivery. It should also be clear to patients that they will be paying a higher cost for IVF if they in fact succeed on the first or second cycle than if they had not chosen the risk-sharing program, and that, in any event, the costs of screening and drugs are not included.

"The Committee was especially concerned about the incentives that risk-sharing programs create for providers to take actions that might harm patients in order to achieve success and avoid a refund. For risk-sharing programs to be ethical, it is imperative that patients be aware of this potential conflict of interest, and that risk-sharing programs not overstimulate patients to obtain a large supply of eggs or transfer more embryos than is safe for the patient, fetus, and prospective offspring. Patients should be fully informed of the risks of multifetal gestation for mother and fetus, and have had ample time to discuss and consider them prior to egg retrieval."

20. Will my insurance pay for my fertility treatments?

Insurance coverage for infertility varies widely across the United States. Several states, including Massachusetts, Illinois, and Maryland, have passed legislative mandates for infertility coverage. In these states, access to fertility treatment is guaranteed through the patient's employer. In the vast majority of states, however, fertility coverage is inconsistent. Some companies may offer extensive fertility benefits, while others offer no coverage at all to their employees.

It is important that you understand your specific benefits before you seek out any kind of fertility treatment. Insurance plans may provide a specific dollar amount to spend on fertility treatments or cover a certain number of cycles of either IUI or IVF. You should work with your fertility provider's billing staff to determine which benefits are available to you before launching into a treatment plan. Given that some insurance plans may cover infertility more extensively than others, it is always appropriate to examine your insurance options during periods of open enrollment for health benefits. Many insurance companies will not cover fertility treatments in patients who have been voluntarily sterilized (e.g., **vasectomy, tubal ligation**). Plans may also have specific requirements in terms of duration of fertility and exclusion criteria for IVF concerning ovarian reserve testing or age.

Vasectomy

Surgical sterilization of a man by cutting the vas deferens.

Tubal ligation

Surgical sterilization of a woman, performed by cutting or occluding the fallopian tubes.

PART THREE

Specific Problems: Polycystic Ovarian Syndrome (PCOS)

What prevents a woman from ovulating normally?

What is polycystic ovarian syndrome?

Where does PCOS come from, and how is it treated?

More . . .

21. What prevents a woman from ovulating normally?

Regular ovulation is associated with regular menstrual cycles. Predictable monthly periods result from the release of an egg 2 weeks prior to the shedding of the endometrial lining of the uterus and in the absence of pregnancy.

If a woman has irregular and unpredictable cycles, then she probably is not ovulating normally. Ovulatory problems are usually divided into two main categories: problems with the ovary and problems with the signals from the brain to the ovary. If a woman's irregular cycles result from a lack of follicles within her ovary, then the failure of the ovary to respond will cause the pituitary gland to secrete increased amounts of follicle-stimulating hormone (FSH). Women with elevated levels of FSH are described as having diminished ovarian reserve; if their periods cease entirely, then they are described as having **premature ovarian failure (POF)**. Different laboratories may vary as to how they define an "elevated" level of FSH, so a discussion with your physician is crucial to correctly assess the results of this test. In most cases, however, an FSH level of more than 15 IU/L is evidence of diminished ovarian reserve; FSH levels exceeding 30 IU/L usually signify POF.

If a woman has a normal complement of follicles but still does not have normal cycles, then the problem must lie elsewhere. Most such women suffer from a communication mismatch between the brain and ovary, which disrupts the carefully coordinated hormone signals that induce the growth of ovarian follicles. The causes of this disruption can be further classified, with most patients being found to have polycystic ovarian syndrome (see Question 22) as opposed to other hormonal imbalances.

Premature ovarian failure (POF)

Irregular or absent menstrual cycles before the age of 40 years old, resulting from a marked loss of ovarian follicles as evidenced by a high blood level of follicle-stimulating hormone (FSH > 30 IU).

If a woman has irregular and unpredictable cycles, then she probably is not ovulating normally.

22. What is polycystic ovarian syndrome?

Polycystic ovarian syndrome (PCOS) is an exceedingly common reproductive disorder, affecting an estimated 10% to

15% of reproductive-age women. The diagnosis of PCOS is a clinical one. In 2003, the ESHRE/ASRM consensus conference redefined PCOS as the presence of at least two out of the three following clinical criteria:

1. Irregular menstrual cycles
2. Evidence of extra male hormones, as determined either by clinical examination or by blood tests
3. Ultrasound demonstrating ovaries with numerous small follicles (PCO-appearing ovaries)

Previously, only patients with irregular menstrual cycles were thought to have PCOS, so the expansion of this definition has led to some confusion among healthcare providers. Other features commonly associated with PCOS include obesity, **insulin resistance**, borderline diabetes, skin tags, and a velvety discoloration on the nape of the neck and inner thighs called **acanthosis nigricans**.

Insulin resistance

Impaired response to insulin, which can lead eventually to diabetes.

Acanthosis nigricans

A velvety skin discoloration associated with insulin resistance.

Kristin comments:

Looking back at my early menstrual cycles, it should have come as no surprise that my reproductive system was not in normal working order. I had extremely heavy periods, but they were never regular. Sometimes I would go months without a period. I didn't think much about it until my husband and I started trying to get pregnant. I went off the pill and got a period about 2 months later. I began charting my basal body temperature and discovered that I was not ovulating. I decided to be proactive and saw my OB, who confirmed that I have PCOS. This diagnosis was further confirmed at my first RE visit. The doctor did a transvaginal ultrasound, which showed that both of my ovaries were covered with many small follicles. I did meet the clinical criteria for diagnosing PCOS, but I did not exhibit any of the outwardly apparent features—obesity, skin tags, acanthosis nigricans.

23. Where does PCOS come from, and how is it treated?

The topic of PCOS can fill an entire book. In fact, several books have been devoted to this subject. Although this condition was originally described by Drs. Stein and Leventhal in 1935, our understanding of PCOS has advanced significantly in the last decade.

Originally, PCOS was thought to be an anatomical problem in which a thickened coating around the ovary prevented ovulation. It is now agreed that PCOS represents a hormonal imbalance.

PCOS represents a hormonal imbalance.

At the heart of this disorder is insulin resistance. Insulin is a hormone secreted by the pancreas that induces your body to store the sugar circulating in the bloodstream. Individuals who fail to produce insulin as a result of an autoimmune disorder require insulin therapy to maintain normal blood sugar levels. These patients are referred to as having insulin-dependent diabetes (also known as type 1 diabetes).

The majority of patients with impaired glucose metabolism actually suffer from insulin resistance rather than insulin deficiency. That is, the cells of their bodies are not sensitive to the effects of insulin, so they require ever-increasing amounts of insulin to be released from the pancreas until appropriate blood levels of glucose are obtained. These patients are commonly referred to as having non-insulin-dependent diabetes (also known as type 2 diabetes or adult-onset diabetes). Despite the name of the disease, persons with type 2 diabetes may require insulin injections to maintain normal glucose levels depending on their degree of insulin resistance.

Insulin resistance is often a genetic disorder. This explains why adult-onset type 2 diabetes is so prevalent in certain families and in certain ethnic groups. In patients who are insulin resistant, the excessive levels of insulin affect not only their metabolism, but also their reproductive system. Insulin directly affects the release of reproductive hormones from the pituitary gland and directly stimulates ovarian production of male hormones. Thus the presence of excess insulin results in a local environment that is not conducive to follicle growth. When multiple follicles fail to grow, they release excessive male hormones, resulting in the acne and abnormal hair growth commonly encountered in women with PCOS. Obesity itself also increases insulin resistance, so patients can find themselves trapped in a vicious cycle of irregular cycles and worsening weight gain. Women who have always had regular periods during their entire life but suddenly gain significant weight can find themselves resembling patients with PCOS. In these cases weight loss by itself may restore normal cycles and improve fertility.

Weight loss by itself may restore normal cycles and improve fertility.

24. If I have PCOS, why do I need to take metformin? Isn't that a drug for diabetics?

The role of insulin resistance as the probable initiating factor in PCOS has important clinical implications. Because of the pioneering work done by Drs. John Nestler and Andrea Dunaif, the treatment of patients with PCOS has now shifted toward addressing the underlying issue of insulin resistance. Patients with PCOS are often treated with an insulin-sensitizing medication such as metformin (Glucophage). Approximately 20% of patients with PCOS and irregular cycles will experience a restoration of their normal cycles with metformin treatment. Because most patients who take metformin experience a diminished appetite, they may also benefit from weight loss with this therapy. Patients with PCOS also have increased rates of first-trimester miscarriage, and preliminary data suggest that there is a reduced rate of miscarriage in patients with PCOS who are treated with metformin.

The dose of metformin is increased gradually. Many physicians initially prescribe 500 mg a day of the extended-release preparation of metformin, to be taken at dinner. After 1 week, the dose is increased to 1000 mg; after another week, the dose is increased to the maximum of 1500 mg. Most patients can tolerate the medication, although severe gastrointestinal side effects (mainly diarrhea) arise in 10% to 15% of patients. Patients who fail to resume predictable cycles with metformin therapy alone will need to consider ovulation induction with fertility medications.

The use of metformin as a first-line medication in the treatment of ovulation problems in patients with PCOS is controversial. Some physicians believe that clomiphene should be the first medication prescribed to women with PCOS who desire pregnancy and have irregular cycles. Our preference has been to start with metformin and then add clomiphene if a women fails to resume regular menstrual cycles.

Kristin comments:

My OB suggested I try metformin to regulate my cycles. I started on 500 mg and eventually went up to 1000 mg—and it worked. I started to get regular periods. By charting my basal body temperature, I could tell that I was ovulating. I experienced major gastrointestinal issues with the drug, but they subsided after a month or so with some flare-ups on occasion. The side effects were worth it as far as I was concerned, especially if the metformin was going to help me get pregnant. When I started seeing an RE, my metformin dose was upped to 1500 mg. Once I did get pregnant through IVF, I remained on metformin for the first trimester of my pregnancy.

> *Patients who fail to resume predictable cycles with metformin therapy alone will need to consider ovulation induction with fertility medications.*

25. I have PCOS and am still not having normal cycles with metformin. What comes next?

Patients who fail to respond to metformin may require ovulation induction with either clomiphene citrate (Clomid) or injectable fertility medications (**gonadotropins**).

Gonadotropins
Fertility medications containing follicle-stimulating hormone alone or in combination with luteinizing hormone.

Clomid has been an FDA-approved treatment for **anovulation** since the late 1960s. This anti-estrogen has been used successfully in millions of women with few complications. Clomid binds to estrogen receptors in the brain, causing the pituitary gland to resume normal release of FSH, and thereby inducing follicles to grow and ultimately release an egg. Patients should take the lowest effective dose of Clomid needed to induce ovulation. With increasing doses, the anti-estrogen side effects can reduce fertility by altering the cervical mucus and leading to a thinner endometrial lining. Many physicians initially prescribe a dose of 50 mg of Clomid to be taken on cycle days 5 to 9. The physician may perform ultrasound monitoring after day 12. Most patients will ovulate around day 17. If no dominant follicle emerges by this day, then an increased dose of 100 mg should be used in the next cycle. A dose of 150 mg is rarely prescribed, because the vast majority of Clomid-responsive patients will ovulate while taking the 50- or 100-mg dose.

Women with PCOS who fail to respond to Clomid can be treated with injectable fertility medications. Gonadotropins are prepared either using recombinant DNA technology (Follistim, Gonal-F) or by isolating these hormones from the urine of postmenopausal women (Bravelle, Menopur). By following a very-low-dose protocol (37.5 IU as the starting dose), approximately 90% of patients will achieve a single dominant follicle. If the treatment produces multiple follicles, however, the woman's risk of multiple pregnancy and **ovarian hyperstimulation syndrome (OHSS)** may lead to cycle cancellation. Almost all of the high-order multiple pregnancies (e.g., sextuplets) born today result from PCOS patients who took gonadotropins and demonstrated an excessive follicular response.

Anovulation

Failure to release an egg on a regular basis, resulting in irregular or absent periods.

Ovarian hyperstimulation syndrome (OHSS)

Ovarian enlargement, abdominal fluid retention, and dehydration following the use of fertility medication to induce the growth of multiple follicles.

Women with PCOS who fail to respond to Clomid can be treated with injectable fertility medications (gonadotropins).

26. If I don't have either PCOS or POF, then what is my problem and why am I not ovulating?

Hormone abnormalities other than PCOS can also lead to irregular menstrual cycles. Such abnormalities include problems with the thyroid gland (which produces a hormone that controls metabolism), abnormal levels of prolactin (a hormone that induces breast milk production), and a lack of pituitary stimulation to the ovary known as **functional hypothalamic amenorrhea (FHA)**. The pituitary gland has been called the master gland of the body; it secretes hormones that control a wide range of functions, including reproduction, metabolism, response to stress, water balance, and growth.

Women with irregular cycles should have their thyroid hormone and prolactin levels measured, because problems with the thyroid gland can indirectly lead to elevations in prolactin. Low levels of thyroid hormone (hypothyroidism) and elevations in prolactin (**hyperprolactinemia**) can be readily treated with medication. In fact, treatment of hypothyroidism with oral thyroid hormone (levothyroxine) can promptly restore normal menstruation. Similarly, hyperprolactinemia usually responds quickly to bromocriptine therapy, often promptly restoring normal cycles.

An elevation of prolactin in the absence of any thyroid disease requires magnetic resonance imaging (MRI) of the brain to evaluate its cause. In such cases, hyperprolactinemia usually results from an increased growth of the prolactin-secreting cells in the pituitary gland that forms a small tumor. If the prolactin-secreting tumor is less than 1 cm in diameter, then it is called a **microadenoma**. A whereas a **macroadenoma** is greater than 1 cm in diameter.

Women without thyroid or prolactin issues who fail to have menstrual periods following treatment with progesterone are usually referred to as having functional hypothalamic amen-

Functional hypothalamic amenorrhea (FHA)

The absence of menstrual cycles related to failure of the hypothalamus and pituitary gland to stimulate follicular growth.

Hyperprolactinemia

Excessive secretion of the hormone prolactin.

Microadenoma

A tumor of the pituitary gland measuring less than 1 cm.

Macroadenoma

A tumor of the pituitary gland measuring more than 1 cm.

Osteoporosis

Loss of calcium and bone mass, leading to an increased risk of fracture.

orrhea (FHA). These women fail to produce normal levels of estrogen despite an appropriate complement of ovarian follicles. Women who are below ideal body weight and who exercise frequently and vigorously are particularly prone to developing this problem. Women with FHA are at risk for **osteoporosis** and should discuss with their physician the benefits of hormone therapy (such as oral contraceptives) when not attempting pregnancy. They should also undergo an MRI of the brain to rule out any structural etiology for their condition. Women who are below ideal body weight may resume normal menstrual cycles when they gain weight or decrease their exercise frequency and duration.

Infertility in women with FHA can be readily treated with injectible gonadotropins. In such women, the choice of medication is important as the drug should contain both FSH and L (Menopur) and not just FSH alone (Gonal-F, Follistim). Clomid rarely works in women with FHA, but nearly all women with FHA can undergo successful ovulation induction.

Specific Problems: Polycystic Ovarian Syndrome

PART FOUR

Specific Problems: Tubal Disease

Can fallopian tubes be repaired?

Why should blocked fallopian tubes be repaired
before IVF is attempted?

If I had my tubes tied, can I have them untied?

More . . .

27. Can fallopian tubes be repaired?

Prior to the advent of IVF, surgical repair of damaged fallopian tubes was considered standard medical care. Unfortunately, most patients did not become pregnant following this procedure, and 10% to 20% experienced tubal (ectopic) pregnancies. Today, IVF has replaced reparative tubal surgery for most patients with damaged fallopian tubes for two reasons: (1) IVF is a nonsurgical treatment and (2) it results in excellent pregnancy rates, especially for patients with tubal disease.

Some patients ask, "Why is it so difficult to repair damaged tubes?" Unfortunately, the problems that cause tubal disease, such as pelvic infections, usually damage the tubal **fimbria**—that is, the delicate finger-like projections at the end of the tube that are responsible for capturing the egg when it is released from the ovary. Pelvic infections may also damage the tubal muscle and inner mucosa, leaving behind a scarred, nonfunctional organ that is not amenable to surgical repair.

In general, most patients with tubal disease are best treated using IVF. Tubal reparative surgery is usually not effective and, in fact, it may increase the woman's risk for having an ectopic or tubal pregnancy. If a couple is not interested in IVF or if they are not deemed to be good candidates for IVF, then tubal surgery may be the only option available to them in terms of fertility treatment.

28. Why should blocked fallopian tubes be repaired before IVF is attempted?

When the fimbria of the fallopian tubes become damaged, it may result in a tube that is blocked at the very distal end—the part farthest away from the uterus. If the tube then becomes filled with fluid, it is called a **hydrosalpinx** ("hydro" refers to water; "salpinx" refers to the fallopian tube itself).

Fimbria

The finger-like projections at the distal end of the fallopian tube that are responsible for trapping the egg following ovulation.

Most patients with tubal disease are best treated using IVF.

Hydrosalpinx

Obstruction of the fallopian tube at the fimbria, resulting in a fluid-filled and dilated tube.

Women who have a hydrosalpinx should have their fallopian tubes either removed or cut prior to undergoing IVF. The surgery usually involves a simple outpatient procedure called laparoscopy. The tubes are cut or removed so that the tubal fluid, which would be toxic to an embryo or adversely affect the receptivity of the endometrial lining, does not flow backward into the uterine cavity, preventing implantation of the embryo.

It is now well recognized that women with an untreated hydrosalpinx have a substantially reduced chance for pregnancy with IVF. In addition, an untreated hydrosalpinx may increase the chance that a woman will experience a spontaneous abortion or miscarriage. For all these reasons, treating a hydrosalpinx should both increase the IVF pregnancy rate and decrease the chances for an early pregnancy loss. A patient with a single normal fallopian tube and a hydrosalpinx will also have a higher chance of achieving a spontaneous pregnancy after removal or ligation of the damaged tube.

It is now well recognized that women with an untreated hydrosalpinx have a substantially reduced chance for pregnancy with IVF.

A hydrosalpinx, if present, is usually identified during the infertility diagnostic evaluation with a hysterosalpingogram (HSG). This simple x-ray study should be performed in all infertile women unless a diagnostic laparoscopy has already been performed. Preoperatively, we advise all patients that we recommend removal or ligation of her tube(s) if a hydrosalpinx is discovered at laparoscopy.

29. If I had my tubes tied, can I have them untied?

Fertile women who have had their "tubes tied" (tubal ligation) may do very well and achieve pregnancy with tubal reparative surgery. Pregnancy rates of 70% to 80% are noted in women who undergo a tubal reversal procedure, depending on their age, the type of tubal ligation procedure performed, and the presence (or absence) of other infertility factors.

Most often, this repair (**tubal reanastamosis**) requires a laparotomy, which involves opening of the abdomen. This major surgery requires 2 to 4 weeks for recovery, and most insurers do not cover it. Some physicians have reported good success with laparoscopic tubal reanastamosis, but this approach can be more technically challenging. As a consequence, most female patients choose to undergo a nonsurgical IVF procedure instead. Studies have shown that IVF is usually more cost-effective than surgical reanastomosis of the fallopian tubes. Specifically, if the surgery fails to establish a pregnancy, then IVF may be necessary anyway.

30. If I had a previous ectopic pregnancy, what should I do to avoid another one?

The reported incidence of tubal or ectopic pregnancy in the general population is 1%. Women who have experienced an ectopic pregnancy generally have a 10% to 15% risk for another ectopic pregnancy. The good news is that most women who have had an ectopic pregnancy will not have another one. The bad news is there are no therapies available to eliminate this risk. All women who are attempting to conceive inherently are at risk for an ectopic pregnancy. Even women with absent or obstructed fallopian tubes can experience an ectopic pregnancy if the embryo becomes implanted in the section of the fallopian tube found within the muscle of the uterus (called an interstitial or cornual pregnancy). The rate of ectopic pregnancy following IVF is usually 1% to 2%, far lower than the 15% recurrence risk with a spontaneous pregnancy.

Women who have experienced an ectopic pregnancy generally have a 10% to 15% risk for another ectopic pregnancy.

Fortunately, most ectopic pregnancies are readily diagnosed very early in pregnancy using blood hormone assays for beta **human chorionic gonadotropin (HCG)** combined with transvaginal ultrasonography. It is now uncommon for such pregnancies to go undiagnosed or to lead to tubal rupture, hemorrhage, or death. Most ectopic pregnancies can be treated medically using low doses of methotrexate (a type of chemotherapy that selectively destroys the pregnancy tissue), thereby avoiding surgery. This medical therapy is 80% to 95% effective.

Kristin comments:

I had an ectopic pregnancy after a Clomid cycle that was monitored by my OB. I was 8 to 9 weeks pregnant and thought I was having a miscarriage when the ectopic pregnancy was confirmed at my first RE appointment. Unfortunately, the methotrexate therapy did not work, and I had to have surgery to remove my right fallopian tube. After determining that my remaining tube was not blocked through an HSG, and with the counsel of our new RE, we opted to move on to IVF. This option would offer the greatest chance for us to become pregnant and avoid another ectopic pregnancy.

When I did become pregnant through IVF, my RE agreed to a very early ultrasound to make sure that the pregnancy was in my uterus. I appreciated that my RE understood my concerns of having another ectopic pregnancy. He treated me as an individual instead of requiring me to wait until the typical 7-week mark to perform an ultrasound.

PART FIVE

Specific Problems: Male Factor

Can surgery improve sperm quality?

Is there anything my husband can do to improve his sperm count, such as wearing boxers and not briefs or taking vitamins?

What can cause my husband to have no sperm at all?

More . . .

31. Can surgery improve sperm quality?

Varicocelectomy

Ligation of dilated testicular or inguinal veins thought to be a source of male infertility.

Varicocele

One or more dilated veins often located in the scrotal sac and thought to be a possible cause of male infertility.

Surgical treatments for male factor infertility are very limited. Historically, **varicocelectomy** has been the surgical procedure most commonly used to improve sperm quality. In this procedure, dilated veins in the scrotum (**varicocele**) are cut or ligated. One theory is that these dilated veins may increase the scrotal-testicular temperature, thereby diminishing the sperm quality. By cutting the veins, the scrotal temperature is restored to normal and fecundity may be improved.

Unfortunately, well-designed controlled studies have not shown any statistical increase in pregnancy rates following varicocelectomy. Furthermore, many fertile men have varicoceles. Today, this procedure is rarely, if ever, indicated. In most cases of male factor infertility, the best treatment involves intrauterine insemination (IUI) or, more often, proceeding directly with in vitro fertilization (IVF) and possibly intracytoplasmic sperm injection (ICSI).

32. Is there anything my husband can do to improve his sperm count, such as wearing boxers and not briefs or taking vitamins?

Sperm parameters demonstrate considerable variation from sample to sample.

Sperm parameters demonstrate considerable variation from sample to sample, so researchers have not been able to identify any specific diet or lifestyle change that might potentially improve sperm quality. Although the presence of a varicocele has been suggested to play a role in male infertility (see Question 31), the benefit of varicocelectomy remains controversial.

Some studies have suggested that wearing boxers instead of briefs can improve a man's sperm count. The avoidance of extremely high temperature may also improve sperm counts, so care should be taken to avoid prolonged exposure to extremely high temperatures, such as within a sauna or a hot tub.

The effects of a variety of nutritional supplements on semen have been studied. Some researchers have suggested that antioxidants may improve sperm quality, thereby leading to improved pregnancy rates (the desired outcome). Although the data on nutritional supplements with antioxidant properties are somewhat limited, a commercially available product based on this research is available (Proxeed, Sigma-Tau Pharmaceuticals). This nutritional supplement is available for purchase only over the Internet. Although it has been frequently prescribed by some urologists, additional studies are required to confirm its benefits.

33. What can cause my husband to have no sperm at all?

Assuming that there was not a problem in collecting the specimen, the absence of sperm on a semen analysis—a condition known as **azoospermia**—requires thorough evaluation. Azoospermia can be divided into two major categories: obstructive and nonobstructive.

Obstructive azoospermia occurs when the duct carrying the sperm from the testicle to the urethra becomes blocked. This blockage may be the result of previous surgery on the scrotum or testicle, or even follow repair of an inguinal hernia. During such surgery, the vas deferens may have been inadvertently damaged or even cut. Scar tissue can also form either postoperatively or following an infection (most commonly gonorrhea, though other infectious diseases may also cause blockage of the sperm duct).

Some men are born without a vas deferens on either side. This **congenital bilateral absence of the vas deferens (CBAVD)** is associated with the gene for cystic fibrosis. In other words, CBAVD is a rather unusual presentation of cystic fibrosis that occurs in the absence of any chronic lung disease. For this reason, any man with azoospermia associated with congenital absence of the vas deferens should undergo genetic testing to determine whether he carries the gene that causes cystic fibrosis.

Azoospermia
The absence of sperm in a semen analysis.

Azoospermia can be divided into two major categories: obstructive and nonobstructive.

Congenital bilateral absence of the vas deferens (CBAVD)

Absence of the sperm-carrying duct in a man, resulting in azoospermia. This condition is frequently associated with cystic fibrosis.

Nonobstructive azoospermia is the result of a dysfunction in sperm production and can represent a more problematic situation. The source of the production problem may be the result of either a testicular issue or a pituitary or hypothalamus issue causing a failure of sperm production in an otherwise normal testis. If a hormonal evaluation reveals normal levels of prolactin and thyroid hormone, then testicular sperm production may have failed. If this finding is associated with an elevated FSH level, then the chance of finding any sperm production in the testis is quite unlikely. A testicular biopsy can be performed to assess whether any sperm are present within the testis. Even very low levels of sperm production may allow for attempts at IVF using ICSI. Genetic testing to rule out a chromosomal problem is often suggested in cases of very low or absent sperm production.

34. Can men with azoospermia father children?

When the male partner has either obstructive or nonobstructive azoospermia, the use of IVF and ICSI may still enable the couple to successfully achieve pregnancy. Sperm from the testis or **epididymis** are essentially unable to fertilize an egg without ICSI. To obtain sperm for use in IVF, a needle aspiration of the testis or epididymis can be performed under local anesthesia. If the male partner has nonobstructive azoospermia, a urologist usually performs a testicular biopsy in the hospital while the patient is under general anesthesia. In either case, the testicular tissue or the sperm aspirate can be frozen in liquid nitrogen and maintained relatively indefinitely. If a testicular biopsy reveals no mature sperm, then the only option is to use donor sperm or to pursue adoption.

Occasionally, the sperm retrieved in this fashion is of exceedingly poor quality. In such cases, a repeat testicular biopsy on the day of **egg collection** for IVF or even use of a **cryopreserved** specimen from an anonymous sperm donor may be considered as a backup plan.

Epididymis

Paired sac-like structures that are found atop each testicle and that serve as a repository for sperm prior to ejaculation.

When the male partner has either obstructive or nonobstructive azoospermia, the use of IVF and ICSI may still enable the couple to successfully achieve pregnancy.

Egg collection

A minimally invasive procedure usually performed transvaginally under minimal sedation in which eggs are removed from the ovaries.

Cryopreservation

Freezing of sperm, eggs, or embryos so as to preserve them for use at a later date.

Rarely, men with diabetes or those taking certain antihypertensive medications may suffer from **retrograde ejaculation**. In this condition, there is no emission of fluid with male orgasm because all of the fluids travel backward into the bladder instead of out through the urethra. Retrograde ejaculation can easily be diagnosed by checking the post-ejaculation voided urine for sperm. Sperm present in the man's urine can be washed and used for either insemination or IVF. Pretreatment with bicarbonate the night before sperm collection may improve sperm quality by increasing the pH of the urine.

One final (and interesting) cause of azoospermia is anabolic steroid abuse. Some men with azoospermia may have used testosterone or other steroids as part of their strength and conditioning training. High doses of these steroids can suppress sperm production. In such patients, sperm production can be reinitiated by stopping the steroids and placing the men on gonadotropin therapy (analogous to ovulation induction in women). Although clomiphene citrate has been used to improve sperm quality in men, most studies reveal it to have little to no benefit.

35. Should I consider using a sperm donor to conceive?

Couples who desire a child but in whom the male partner has a very low sperm count (**oligospermia**) or no sperm at all (azoospermia) often consider using third-party sperm donation and artificial insemination. Donor sperm can also be used by single women or lesbian couples. Many high-quality, reputable commercial sperm banks exist. They recruit and thoroughly test the donors and provide a listing of their available donors and their characteristics from which the couple can then choose. The donated sperm is obtained from the donor, tested, and quarantined for at least 6 months at the sperm bank. The donors are then retested.

Retrograde ejaculation

Backward movement of semen into the urinary bladder at the time of ejaculation.

Oligospermia

An abnormally low concentration of sperm in a semen analysis.

53

The specimen is released for use only after the tests results are confirmed as normal. The frozen sperm is then usually sent to the physician's office, and artificial insemination is performed around the time of the woman's ovulation. Placement of the sperm inside the uterus (IUI) results in better pregnancy rates than placement of the sperm in the vagina or cervix. Frozen donor sperm can also be used for more advanced fertility procedures such as gonadotropin/IUI or IVF with or without ICSI. If a woman wishes to use sperm from a known donor with whom she does not have a physical relationship, then the sperm may need to be quarantined for at least 6 months and the donor retested for infectious diseases before the specimen can be used for fertility treatments.

PART SIX

Specific Problems: Endometriosis

What is endometriosis and how is it diagnosed?

Does surgery for endometriosis improve pregnancy rates?

Are there medical treatments for endometriosis?

More . . .

36. What is endometriosis and how is it diagnosed?

Endometriosis is the presence of endometrial-like tissue located outside of the uterine cavity. Most commonly, it is located on the ovaries, but it can also be found on any of the organs inside the pelvic–abdominal cavities. Although its etiology is unknown, endometriosis may arise when menstruation is obstructed, resulting in retrograde menstrual flow into the tubes and pelvic cavity. Just as the endometrium bleeds every month during menstruation, so, too, does the ectopically located endometriosis. This phenomenon leads to inflammation of the pelvic reproductive organs, causing pelvic pain, painful periods (**dysmenorrhea**), and infertility. Pelvic adhesions or scar tissue may also develop.

Dysmenorrhea

Extremely painful periods.

Endometriosis may be suspected when patients complain of increasingly severe dysmenorrhea, pelvic pain, or infertility, but it can be definitively diagnosed only via surgery. Most often, a diagnostic laparoscopy—a simple outpatient surgical procedure—is used to diagnose endometriosis. Other nonsurgical techniques such as ultrasonography, CT scan, or MRI can occasionally be helpful in their abilities to detect endometriosis.

Endometriosis can be definitively diagnosed only via surgery.

37. Does surgery for endometriosis improve pregnancy rates?

Well-designed medical studies clearly show that destroying even small amounts of endometriotic tissue can improve fertility by as much as 50%. In a large Canadian study, the monthly pregnancy rate following surgical treatment of minimal endometriosis rose from 3% to 4.5%. Although this finding represented a 50% improvement in the patients' monthly chance of pregnancy, it does not compare very favorably with IVF pregnancy rates, which average around 30% for a single treatment cycle. Nevertheless, because treatment of endometriosis at the time of surgery does improve pregnancy rates, most doctors will destroy the abnormal endometriotic tissue at the time of the diagnostic laparoscopy by using either laser or coagulation techniques. In addition to improving fertility, surgery may often eliminate or improve symptoms of dysmenorrhea and pelvic pain.

Ovarian cysts that contain endometriotic tissue may grow quite large. They are often called "chocolate cysts" because of the dark brown fluid found within them, although endometriosis cysts are more correctly referred to as **endometriomas**. If left untreated, these growths may destroy part or all of the normal ovarian tissue, including the eggs. Endometriomas must be surgically removed, usually via laparoscopy. Sometimes, however, laparotomy is required. The ultimate choice of which surgery is performed depends on the operative findings and the skill and experience of the surgeon. Medical treatment of endometriomas is insufficient and will not cause these cysts to resolve.

38. Are there medical treatments for endometriosis?

Several medications exist to treat endometriosis. All of them are designed to suppress the endometriotic implants by suppressing ovulation and causing a **hypoestrogenic** state. Unfortunately, suppressing ovulation also prevents pregnancy from occurring. In patients who are not trying to conceive, medical treatment of endometriosis can be very beneficial and relieve symptoms of dysmenorrhea and pelvic pain.

One common medical treatment involves **oral contraceptive pills** taken on a daily basis. Although each of these pills contains estrogen, the progestin (progesterone-like component) in the pill overrides the estrogen effect, resulting in suppression of the endometriotic lesions. Oral contraceptive pills are effective in 30% to 60% of patients with endometriosis-related pain.

Endometriomas

An ovarian cyst that is filled with chocolate-colored fluid as a result of endometriosis growing within the ovary.

Hypoestrogenic:

A state of low estrogen.

Oral contraceptive pills

Daily medications, usually containing both synthetic estrogen and progesterone, that act as very effective contraceptives by suppressing follicle growth and ovulation.

Gonadotropin-releasing hormone (GnRH) analog

Medication that initially causes the pituitary gland to release its stores of follicle-stimulating hormone and luteinizing hormone, but that with continued use leads to markedly suppressed levels of these two hormones.

Many physicians prescribe **gonadotropin-releasing hormone (GnRH) analogs** (such as Lupron), which reduce estrogen levels to postmenopausal levels for their patients with endometriosis. These medications suppress estrogen production, prevent ovulation, and cause atrophy of the endometriosis in 70% to 90% patients. Unfortunately, GnRH analogs are expensive and must be given as injections either once a month or every 3 months. GnRH agonists can cause side effects including headaches, hot flashes, moodiness, insomnia, and vaginal dryness.

To counteract these problems, physicians often prescribe oral contraceptive pills or supplemental progestin therapy such as norethindrone along with the GnRH analogs. This combined therapy has many advantages, including improved treatment acceptance and alleviation of the many side effects associated with the use of the GnRH analogs as single therapy. Patients tolerate this combination very well and achieve maximal benefits in suppressing the disease and its symptoms.

For patients with endometriosis who are actively trying to conceive, medical therapy is not indicated, because all of these treatments will suppress ovulation. Instead, for these patients, the goal should be to promptly establish pregnancy before the endometriosis causes any further damage to the reproductive organs. Generally, these women should seek treatment from a fertility expert to maximize their chances for successful pregnancy.

For patients with endo-metriosis who are actively trying to conceive, medical therapy is not indicated.

39. Do I need endometriosis surgery if I am already planning to pursue IVF?

This is a somewhat controversial area of reproductive medicine. Most reproductive endocrinologists do not recommend surgery prior to IVF unless the woman has advanced endometriosis, such as an ovarian endometrioma.

For women who have only mild to moderate endometriosis, IVF is associated with excellent pregnancy rates even without surgery. When advanced endometriosis is present, such as an ovarian endometrioma, its surgical removal prior to IVF may enhance the chances for a successful IVF outcome and may decrease infectious complications related to egg collection. Thus, in such cases, most reproductive endocrinologists routinely recommend the removal of advanced endometriosis prior to treatment using IVF.

However, severe endometriosis with endometriomas may lead to diminished ovarian responsiveness, and ovarian surgery may further compromise fertility in such cases. So the decision to perform extensive surgery for endometriosis must be weighed against the potential impact of that surgery on the ovary. Also, advanced endometriosis may increase the likelihood for an early pregnancy loss or spontaneous abortion. By first removing the endometriosis, the outcome of pregnancy may be greatly improved.

PART SEVEN

Treatment Options: Intrauterine Insemination (IUI)

What is the difference (if any) between intrauterine insemination and artificial insemination?

How do I know if IUI is an option for me?

What fertility drugs are used with IUI, and why are they used if I already have normal periods?

More . . .

40. What is the difference (if any) between intrauterine insemination and artificial insemination?

Artificial insemination (AI) is a historical term that encompasses any technique involving the introduction of sperm into the female reproductive tract without sexual intercourse. Semen can be placed into the vagina (intravaginal insemination) or into the cervix (intracervical insemination) without any special preparation of the specimen. However, if unprepared semen is placed directly into the uterus [intrauterine insemination (IUI)], then severe spasmodic uterine cramping can occur. Thus, when performing an IUI, the sperm must first be washed and prepared prior to placement inside the uterus. Washing the sperm removes prostaglandins, the hormones that cause the violent uterine contractions. Washing also eliminates substances that might lower the sperm quality, thereby leading to improved sperm motility. Generally, the IUI specimen is prepared in the doctor's office just prior to insemination.

When performing an IUI, the sperm must first be washed.

The actual IUI is a painless, simple, in-office procedure that is often performed by a nurse. It usually takes just a minute to perform. Physicians typically ask patients to come in with a full bladder so that the angle between the uterus and cervix is altered, which allows for easy passage of the catheter into the uterine cavity.

Today, it is rare for patients to undergo other forms of insemination besides IUI because the pregnancy rates with IUI are better than those obtained by intravaginal insemination or **intracervical insemination**.

Intracervical insemination

A fertility treatment in which sperm are placed within the cervix.

41. How do I know if IUI is an option for me?

IUI is a good option for many infertile couples. It can be performed in conjunction with a woman's natural cycle or can be combined with the use of fertility drugs. IUI can also be effectively used in couples who have sexual dysfunction or infrequent coitus for either medical or nonmedical reasons. For example, some couples may have busy work schedules such that one or the other partner is frequently out of town around the time of ovulation. If the male partner's sperm is obtained and cryopreserved (frozen) in advance of ovulation, the physician (or nurse) can perform an IUI and, ideally, facilitate pregnancy without the woman missing a menstrual cycle.

The best candidates for IUI are those couples without tubal disease (female partner) or severe male factor infertility (male partner). Women with severe endometriosis or a history of pelvic adhesions are not good candidates for IUI. Although couples with male factor infertility can attempt IUI, the success rates are fairly low in such cases, and prompt consideration should be given to IVF (and ICSI) if pregnancy fails to occur after three or four attempts.

42. Which fertility drugs are used with IUI, and why are they used if I already have normal periods?

IUI can produce fair success rates when combined with fertility drugs. Many studies show superior pregnancy rates when IUI is combined with either Clomid or injectable gonadotropins, as compared to using these medications alone. For this reason, most infertility experts will recommend IUI to their patients when treating them with fertility drugs.

In women who fail to ovulate regularly, the goal of drug therapy is to induce the growth and release of a single mature egg. This treatment is known as ovulation induction. In contrast, the treatment goal for women with regular menstrual cycles is to induce the growth of multiple follicles with the subsequent release of multiple eggs. Hence the term **superovulation** (also called **controlled ovarian hyperstimulation**) is used to describe this situation. During a cycle of superovulation and

Superovulation

The development of multiple ovarian follicles in response to fertility medication.

Controlled ovarian hyperstimulation

Stimulation of the ovaries with fertility medications to help them grow and release multiple eggs.

IUI, the goal is to develop 3 to 5 mature follicles, whereas the goal in an IVF cycle is to produce more.

Clomid is the fertility drug of first choice for both ovulation induction and superovulation with IUI. Women who fail to respond to Clomid or who fail to conceive may be candidates for treatment with injectable fertility medications (gonadotropins) combined with IUI. In some cases, it is best to skip the treatment with Clomid and instead proceed directly with gonadotropin therapy; this decision depends on the severity of the couple's infertility situation.

In women who have normal menstrual cycles, it would appear on the surface that IUI alone without fertility drugs would be as successful as IUI with fertility drugs. Unfortunately, this simply is not the case. Instead, the combination of IUI and fertility drugs to induce superovulation yields a synergistic benefit over either treatment alone.

The combination of IUI and fertility drugs to induce superovulation yields a synergistic benefit over either treatment alone.

43. What are typical pregnancy rates for IUI?

The pregnancy rates for IUI vary widely, depending mostly on the female partner's age and the presence or absence of any other infertility factors. In patients younger than 35 years old, an estimated one-third to one-half of patients will achieve pregnancy within 1 to 4 treatments. In patients with unexplained infertility, most studies demonstrate a per-cycle pregnancy rate of 6% for the Clomid/IUI combination and 9% to 12% for the gonadotropin/IUI combination, compared with a spontaneous pregnancy rate of less than 5% per month (see Table 3). Many fertility doctors will try 1 to 4 cycles of Clomid/IUI and then 1 to 4 cycles of gonadotropin/IUI. If pregnancy has not occurred after the fourth treatment, most experts would abandon these treatments and proceed with more aggressive therapy such as in vitro fertilization. The optimal number of IUI treatment cycles should be individually determined by the patient and her infertility specialist.

Table 3   Unexplained Infertility Success Rates Per Cycle with Various Treatment Options

Method	Pregnancy Rate (%)
Intercourse	4
IUI	4
CC	5.6
CC + IUI	8
FSH	7.7
FSH + IUI	17
In vitro fertilization	21

CC, clomiphene citrate; FSH, follicle-stimulating hormone; IUI, intrauterine insemination.
Source: Adapted from Guzick DS, et al. Efficacy of treatment for unexplained infertility. *Fertil Steril* 70:207, 1998.

Some patients develop a seeming resistance to fertility medications, demonstrating reduced responses with repeated stimulations. This problem is especially prevalent in women who are more than 37 years old. Thus IVF should be considered as a first-line treatment in these patients as opposed to multiple gonadotropin/IUI cycles.

44. How many office visits are required during a typical cycle using fertility drugs and IUI?

For treatments using Clomid and IUI, only a couple of office visits per month are required. At a typical office visit, the patient has her blood drawn for hormone analysis, and a pelvic ultrasound is performed to measure the size of the follicles. The doctor uses this information to determine the optimal timing of the HCG trigger shot and the subsequent IUI.

For treatment using gonadotropins and IUI, closer monitoring is necessary, perhaps requiring 4 to 6 office visits per treatment cycle. The actual IUI takes only minutes to perform and is usually painless. We routinely ask our patients to lie on their backs for about 10 to 15 minutes following the IUI procedure. The woman may then return to her normal activities.

45. I read on the Internet that two inseminations are better than one. Is this true?

This is not true. In general, one well-timed IUI is as good as two, and no advantages are obtained by performing a second IUI (providing ovulation was well monitored using blood hormone determinations and follicle ultrasound measurements). However, in patients who are undergoing IUI with less intense monitoring of ovulation, such as urine LH testing, or for those women who chose not to monitor their ovulation at all, two inseminations may be a better option.

Using basal body temperatures as the basis for an IUI's timing is not recommended, because this method cannot prospectively pinpoint the optimal timing of ovulation for an IUI treatment. The rise in basal body temperature occurs after ovulation, so identifying this temperature increase would not help in scheduling an IUI procedure.

Men who have a low sperm count or motility should abstain from sexual relations for 3 to 5 days prior to a planned IUI.

46. Can we have sex during a treatment cycle?

In general, the answer is yes. Many experts, however, recommend no coitus for 2 to 3 days prior to an anticipated IUI to "build up" the male partner's sperm count and volume. Also, some men may experience difficulty producing a specimen if they have recently had coitus. For men who have a low sperm count or motility, it is recommended that they abstain from sexual relations for 3 to 5 days prior to a planned IUI.

47. My doctor wants to use Lupron or Antagon during my IUI cycle. What are these drugs, and why do I need them? I thought they were only for IVF.

These medications can be used to prevent premature ovulation—that is, they can delay ovulation until the optimal follicle size has been reached. Premature ovulation during an IUI cycle can be dealt with by simply adjusting the timing of the IUI. These medications are primarily used in patients undergoing IVF rather than IUI. For most patients undergoing treatment with IUI, Lupron and Antagon are rarely necessary. These drugs are not routinely used unless a patient repeatedly experiences a premature LH surge during the treatment cycle. In such cases, these medications can allow for a more optimal stimulation.

48. What complications can occur after IUI?

It is very rare for any complications to occur after IUI, because it is a simple, in-office, nonsurgical procedure, usually performed by nurses. Some patients may experience mild to moderate uterine cramps when the catheter is placed inside their uterus. These cramps usually last 10 to 15 minutes. Infection rarely occurs (its incidence is less than 1%). Many infertility specialists routinely obtain cervical cultures prior to initiating an IUI cycle, and the culture media used to prepare the IUI specimen commonly contains antibiotics. Occasionally, patients may note some light spotting after placement of the IUI catheter, but this is not an indication of a complication or a problem. Multiple pregnancy can occur in any situation when two or more mature follicles are present at the time of HCG. Your physician should discuss with you the risk of multiple pregnancy in cycles using fertility medication to induce the growth of multiple follicles.

Multiple pregnancy can occur in any situation when two or more mature follicles are present at the time of HCG.

49. How would I know when to pursue more advanced fertility treatments?

The decision to seek out more advanced fertility treatments is a complex question, and multiple factors must be considered when making it. For most couples undergoing treatment with IUI (either alone or with fertility drugs), the best chances for success usually occur within the first four treatment cycles. After that, the likelihood for pregnancy decreases. In many of our patients, we recommend only one or two IUI treatments. If these efforts are unsuccessful, we suggest that the couple proceed with other more aggressive treatments including both natural cycle IVF and traditional IVF using injectible fertility medications.

For some patients, IUI should rarely be utilized. For example, those couples with severe tubal disease, pelvic adhesions, or severe male factor infertility may do best by directly proceeding with IVF as their first treatment option. If an age factor is present or if the couple has prolonged infertility (infertility lasting more than 5 years), we may recommend IVF first, as well.

PART EIGHT

Treatment Options: In Vitro Fertilization (IVF)

What is IVF, and how is it performed?

How do I know if I need IVF?

How successful is IVF?

More . . .

50. What is IVF, and how is it performed?

In vitro fertilization (IVF) was first successfully performed in Oldham, England, in 1978, resulting in the birth of Louise Brown. Since then, more than 1 million children have been born using IVF. The introduction of this technique completely changed—and greatly improved—our ability to treat even the most difficult cases of infertility, many of which were previously untreatable. Although it is clearly not a "cure-all" for infertility, IVF has revolutionized our approach to, and understanding of, the disease called infertility.

IVF literally means "the fertilization of eggs with sperm in the laboratory." An IVF cycle consists of several discrete phases, as detailed in the sections that follow.

PHASE 1: OVARIAN STIMULATION

A woman's ovaries contain thousands of fluid-filled sacs called follicles. Inside each follicle is an egg (or ovum). In a normal reproductive cycle, only a single follicle (and egg) reaches maturity. Although Louise Brown (the world's first IVF baby) was produced in a natural cycle from a single follicle, this form of IVF is less efficient because it often leads to cancelled cycles as a result of premature ovulation prior to the egg collection or the failure to retrieve the single egg that is produced.

The introduction of injectable gonadotropin drugs enabled physicians to increase the efficiency of IVF through the production of multiple mature follicles. Two forms of these medications are used: (1) drugs containing equal parts of the pituitary hormones follicle-stimulating hormone (FSH) or luteinizing hormone (LH) [Menopur] or (2) drugs containing only FSH (Bravelle, Gonal-F, Follistim). Both kinds of medications induce the growth of multiple ovarian follicles, so it is important to monitor the woman's response to them carefully with ultrasound and blood hormone testing.

In vitro fertilization (IVF) was first successfully performed in Oldham, England, in 1978, resulting in the birth of Louise Brown.

Estrogen is produced within each of the developing follicles and induces the growth of the lining of the uterus (endometrium). Unfortunately, the rise in estrogen can also induce the pituitary gland to prematurely trigger ovulation, resulting in the cancellation of an IVF cycle. Two other classes of drugs are used to reduce the chance of this problem occurring during an IVF stimulation: (1) GnRH agonists (such as Lupron and Synarel) and (2) **GnRH antagonists** (such as Centrotide and Antagon) . Lupron (or Synarel) is usually started 1 week prior to the woman's anticipated next menstrual cycle. Given that a patient may have spontaneously conceived during this cycle, all women beginning Lupron are recommended to use a barrier form of contraception.

Approximately 1 week after starting Lupron, the woman should experience a normal menstrual period. An ultrasound exam is performed at the start of this menstrual cycle to examine the ovaries and measure any existing cysts. In some cases, empty follicles from a previous cycle will persist and may influence the response to FSH. If the baseline ultrasound and blood tests are normal, then the patient receives instructions that afternoon as to when and what dose of medication she should take and when she should report back to the office for repeat ultrasound and blood tests.

Patients remain on Lupron to prevent the premature release of the eggs until the end of the stimulation phase. During a typical treatment cycle, they take daily injections for 9 to 12 days before the follicles reach maturity based on their ultrasound results and blood hormone levels. Once the follicles reach a 20- to 24-mm diameter, the woman receives a final injection of human chorionic gonadotropin (HCG; Pregnyl, Profasi) at a precise time. This hormone serves as a trigger to incite the final maturation and release of the egg (ovulation). Ovulation typically occurs about 40 hours after this shot, so the egg collection procedure is scheduled for 34–36 hours after the HCG injection.

Gonadotropin-releasing hormone (GnRH) antagonist

Medication that quickly interferes with the production of follicle-stimulating hormone and luteinizing hormone by the pituitary gland, preventing premature ovulation during a treatment cycle.

Cycles using GnRH antagonists are somewhat different. GnRH antagonists are started several days following the start of ovarian stimulation with gonadotropins. Most clinics add the GnRH antagonist once the largest follicle reaches a diameter of 14 mm. This medication effectively prevents the release of LH from the pituitary within hours of administration. Although many clinics have used GnRH antagonists successfully as part of their IVF stimulation protocols, some studies have demonstrated a trend towards decreased implantation rates in IVF cycles using this class of medications.

PHASE 2: OOCYTE RETRIEVAL

Many physicians perform IVF as an office-based procedure, whereas others utilize a free-standing surgery center. Some programs are located within a hospital. There are advantages and disadvantages to each of these. We prefer to perform the egg collection within our office, as the location and staff are familiar to the patients undergoing the IVF process. We also find that the location of the IVF lab within the office encourages continuous communication between patient, physician, and embryology staff. However, clearly many successful programs utilize a surgery center or a hospital. The use of a hospital setting may allow patients with significant medical conditions (cardiac disease, severe pulmonary disease) to undergo IVF, whereas such patients would be considered an anesthesia risk in the office setting.

Although many patients are nervous about the oocyte retrieval, in fact the vast majority of women find it to be less uncomfortable than some of the screening tests leading up to IVF. The egg collection is performed under light conscious intravenous sedation using a vaginal ultrasound probe with a special needle guide adapter. The needle passes through the side of the vagina into the ovary, and the follicles are easily aspirated. The fluid containing the eggs is then inspected by the **embryologist** using a microscope. Both the eggs and the sperm are then placed together in small plastic dishes contain-

Embryologist

A scientist involved in the fertilization and culture of human eggs and embryos.

ing media and incubated for the next 3 to 5 days. If there is a significant male factor, then ICSI is performed several hours after the egg collection.

PHASE 3: EMBRYO CULTURE

On the day following the egg collection, patients learn how many eggs were fertilized. Remember that although your RE measures all of the follicles during stimulation, mature eggs are usually found only in follicles with a diameter of more than 17 mm. In general, about 70% of the mature eggs will fertilize; unfortunately, some attrition occurs at each point in an IVF cycle so the total number of healthy embryos is often much less than the original number of follicles or eggs.

Three days after the egg collection procedure, the embryos selected for **embryo transfer** will be identified. If the couple is planning a blastocyst transfer, this step occurs on day 5 or 6. Usually your RE will review the quality of the embryos with the embryologist and then discuss with you his or her recommendations regarding the number of embryos to transfer.

On the day following the egg collection, patients learn how many eggs were fertilized.

Embryo transfer

The placement of embryos created via in vitro fertilization into the uterus or, more rarely, the fallopian tube.

Embryos that are not selected for transfer may still be of excellent quality, so they may be candidates for cryopreservation with liquid nitrogen. These frozen embryos can then be replaced into the uterus during a future cycle, eliminating the need for the woman to undergo the entire IVF process of ovarian stimulation and egg collection. There is little benefit to freezing poor-quality embryos, however, because they are unlikely to result in a pregnancy and may not even survive the thawing process.

PHASE 4: EMBRYO TRANSFER

Embryo transfer is one of the most critical aspects of an IVF cycle. During this phase, the embryos are transferred in a procedure similar to an IUI. At our office, we perform our embryo transfers under abdominal ultrasound guidance to ensure the accurate placement of the embryos into the uterus. On the day of embryo transfer, patients are asked to drink 48 ounces of water and keep a full bladder to enable us to visualize the transfer of the embryos.

PHASE 5: POST-TRANSFER AND PREGNANCY

During the 2 weeks after the embryo transfer, patients take supplemental progesterone (shots and suppositories). If a patient's estrogen level drops significantly during the 2 weeks following embryo transfer, the physician may add supplemental estrogen as well.

Two weeks after the transfer, the woman typically undergoes a blood pregnancy test.

Two weeks after the transfer, the woman typically undergoes a blood pregnancy test. Once a pregnancy test is positive, the physician may repeat the test every 2 days until the woman's beta HCG level is high enough to visualize the pregnancy sac on transvaginal ultrasound (the beta HCG level should be more than 2000 IU around 3 to 4 weeks following embryo transfer). A follow-up ultrasound is then performed to confirm fetal cardiac activity. At this point, patients are transferred to their obstetrician/gynecologist for prenatal care.

Carol comments:

Before undergoing IVF, I remember thinking that Phases 1 through 4 would be the hardest part. I was very intimidated by all the drugs and the shots and the egg collection. In reality, it was Phase 5 that was the toughest. I had done everything I could do—mixed the drugs, given the shots, drank the water. Now all that was left was to wait and see if it worked.

One piece of helpful advice I was given was to plan something out of the ordinary during those 2 weeks. Whether it's a vacation with your husband or visiting a relative, introducing anything that is not part of your normal routine is helpful in keeping your mind off of whether or not you're pregnant.

51. How do I know if I need IVF?

Not all patients need IVF or are good candidates for IVF. Thus the answer to this question can be determined only after you undergo a comprehensive infertility evaluation by your reproductive endocrinologist. Nevertheless, some situations clearly require the use of IVF. For example, women with absent or severely damaged fallopian tubes should be treated immediately with IVF. Likewise, IVF should be performed first if the male partner has very poor sperm quality. For other patients, the use of IVF may be less clear-cut, especially given that many different treatment options exist. In such cases, the doctor should discuss with the couple the pros and cons of each option, and then all parties should jointly decide on a treatment plan.

Kristin comments:

After I lost my right fallopian tube to an ectopic pregnancy, we discussed the various ART options with our RE. Due to my PCOS diagnosis as well as having only one tube, my chance of conceiving during an IUI cycle was around 10% at best, whereas my chance of conceiving via IVF was significantly higher than a typical 30-year-old fertile woman's chance. We were eager to start our family and decided to go with the more aggressive treatment because it had a higher success rate. It helped that our insurance covered the procedure. I think it is important to know the success rates for the treatment options your RE suggests. When given the choice between a 10% chance of conceiving through IUI and a more than 50% chance of conceiving through IVF, the choice seemed clear.

52. How successful is IVF?

Overall, the success rates for IVF have improved markedly since 1978 (when Louise Brown was conceived), but success rates vary widely depending on the couple's infertility factors and the clinic performing the IVF procedure. Success rates for U.S. IVF clinics are published on the CDC's website (www.cdc.gov/ART/index.htm). The standardization of clinic

Wyden law

Legislation passed by the U.S. Congress and sponsored by Congressman Ron Wyden that regulates the advertising and reporting of IVF success rates by fertility clinics.

Success rates for U.S. IVF clinics are published on the CDC's website (www. cdc.gov/ART/ index.htm)

success rates evolved from 1994 passage of the Fertility Clinic Success Rate and Certification Act (the so-called **Wyden law**), which seeks to protect U.S. consumers from inflated IVF success rates. Importantly, many subtleties influence clinic-specific IVF pregnancy rates, including patient selection bias (that is, some clinics tend to treat tougher cases, so their success rates might be lower than those of clinics that take only routine cases).

For women younger than 34 years of age, most will achieve pregnancy within one to three treatment cycles; indeed, many succeed in their first attempt. For women older than 35 years, the success rates tend to decrease simply because the aging process affects the quality of these women's eggs. For a detailed discussion of IVF success rates, couples should visit the website for the clinic where they are considering treatment. They should also discuss their specific likelihood of success with their reproductive endocrinologist. IVF pregnancy rates do vary by clinic, so patients should carefully scrutinize their chances for success at the particular clinic rendering treatment.

Carol comments:

This was one part of the process that I found to be a bit more predictable. In both my pregnancies, it took two IVF attempts to achieve a viable pregnancy. As tough as it was after each failed attempt, I tried to take something positive away. For example, after my very first IVF attempt resulted in a chemical pregnancy, I focused on the fact that I now knew an embryo could implant in the lining of my uterus. When I was trying to get pregnant the second time, I did a FET [frozen embryo transfer] with frozen embryos from the previous cycle. Again, it resulted in a chemical pregnancy. Based on that experience, we decided that we would not pursue another FET. I am convinced that maintaining a positive attitude during the process makes a big difference.

53. Are the children born after IVF normal?

The question of the health of children born after advanced fertility treatments is one that has great importance both to the parents and to fertility physicians. In general, the data regarding the outcomes for children born after IVF, either with or without the use of ICSI, have been extremely reassuring.

The problem with these studies remains the identification of an appropriate control group with which to compare the rate of problems found in the children conceived with advanced fertility techniques. Overall, most studies suggest a background risk of birth defects in naturally conceived children of approximately 4% to 5%. However, these couples tend to be younger than the couples undergoing IVF and, by definition, do not suffer from infertility. Although the vast majority of studies suggest no increased risk of anomalies in children conceived after IVF, none of these studies have looked at the rate of congenital anomalies in children conceived naturally but born to parents who suffered infertility that spontaneously resolved without treatment. This group of patients would clearly represent a more appropriate control group with which to compare with patients who seek out advanced fertility treatments.

Recently, a systematic review was conducted in Australia of all studies that had previously examined the possible increased risk to children conceived after treatment with IVF and/or ICSI (Hansen, M. et al, *Human Reproduction.* 20 (2):328–338, 2005). However, many of these studies compare the rate of congenital abnormalities in children conceived spontaneously with the rate in children who were born to older couples undergoing IVF and/or ICSI. In many studies, the rate of congenital anomalies in the control group have been around 4%, whereas the rate of congenital anomalies in the group of couples undergoing IVF and ICSI have been 6% or greater. The difference between 4% and 6% is statistically significant and suggests that there may be an increased risk to children conceived through the use of advanced reproductive techniques. However, the question remains as to whether this is a problem related to IVF itself or to the

The vast majority of studies suggest no increased risk of anomalies in children conceived after IVF.

underlying infertility that leads to the use of IVF. In any case, most patients accept an increased absolute risk of 2% as being reasonable, especially given that their options for spontaneous conception may be significantly limited.

The greatest risk to the children conceived after fertility treatment is that of prematurity related to multiple pregnancy. Several strategies are used to reduce the rate of multiple gestations (see Question 54, which deals with how many embryos to transfer in IVF). The risks of prematurity are significant and should not be discounted quickly, especially given that 50% of twins deliver a month or more before their due date.

The greatest risk to the children conceived after fertility treatment is that of prematurity related to multiple pregnancy.

In addition, the question has been raised as to whether even IVF singleton pregnancies are at higher risk for low birth weight and prematurity. If true, the cause of this increased risk may be difficult to determine. Patients undergoing IVF suffer from infertility, so any increased rate of adverse pregnancy outcome might not be so much a result of the IVF process as it is related to the couple's underlying problem of infertility. Several studies have suggested that women who conceive spontaneously, but who have a preceding history of infertility, have a significantly increased rate of prematurity and pregnancy-related complications such as placenta previa, abruption, and low-birth-weight infants.

Gestational carrier

A woman who undergoes an embryo transfer consisting of an embryo produced by another couple (or from donor gametes) with the intention to give the resulting baby back to the genetic parents.

Another way to look at the question of whether any risk is related to the process of IVF itself versus the patient who is undergoing IVF is to examine the pregnancy outcomes in women who undergo IVF but use a **gestational carrier** (carriers usually have an excellent reproductive history). A study of these pregnancies found there was no increased risk of prematurity or low birth weight in the children conceived and carried in this way. This reassuring outcome would suggest that the problem lies not so much with the IVF process but, unfortunately, with the patients who require IVF to conceive.

The impact of new and emerging technologies on the rate of congenital anomalies in children born after fertility treatment remains a subject of ongoing debate. The potential risks inherent in micromanipulation of the embryo prior to embryo transfer—like that required for preimplantation genetic diagnosis (PGD)—remain unknown. Although more than 3 million IVF babies have been delivered worldwide to date, only a relatively small number of children have been delivered after the use of PGD or following unusual situations such as performing rescue ICSI on the day following egg collection because of unanticipated failed fertilization. When considering such novel treatments, the physician needs to inform the patient /couple of any known or suspected risks. Currently, several studies are under way in this country and throughout the world to continue to monitor the health of those children delivered following advanced fertility treatments.

Carol comments:

Although this question is focused on the "physical normalcy" of IVF babies, I would like to comment on the "perceived normalcy" of IVF babies. I do understand that a large percentage of people will never have to deal with this challenge, and that ignorance is bliss, but I am still surprised by how commonplace the misperceptions related to ART are.

I'll never forget a comment that a woman made to me during my first pregnancy. I was flying back from a visit with my extended family during which we had announced the long-awaited news that I was pregnant. My husband and I struck up a conversation with the woman sitting next to us. As what now seems inevitable, the subject of IVF came up. I confirmed that my pregnancy was, indeed, a result of IVF. Without missing a beat, the woman looked at me and said, "I've never seen one of those babies." I was astounded. Luckily, my husband was there to help me regain my composure and politely explain to the woman that, in fact, IVF babies are not from Mars. Long story short, it's hard to anticipate what people might say to you, so be prepared.

54. How do I decide how many embryos to transfer?

Determining the number of embryos to transfer in an IVF cycle is a crucial decision that requires careful discussion between the patient/couple and the physician. The goal of every treatment cycle should be the delivery of a full-term, healthy, singleton baby. Although transferring more than one embryo will increase the pregnancy rate, at some point transferring additional embryos merely serves to increase the multiple pregnancy rate without altering the overall pregnancy rate. Several European countries have eliminated all discussion of how many embryos to transfer by mandating that all patients undergo only single-embryo transfers. Whereas elective (or mandatory) single-embryo transfer has been promoted heavily throughout Europe, it has not yet received widespread acceptance in the United States.

One of the major disadvantages of single-embryo transfer is that it leads to a decreased IVF pregnancy rate from the fresh cycle. Proponents of single-embryo transfer claim that the potential reduction in the overall pregnancy rate is well worth the marked reduction in the twin pregnancy rate. Twin pregnancies can be problematic because they are associated with higher rates of preterm labor and preterm delivery. Some couples, however, may desire twins or at least regard them as a neutral outcome. This view is especially prevalent among patients who are paying for the treatment themselves (rather than it being covered by insurance) and regard twins as a "two for the price of one" outcome. As noted in Question 53, the greatest risk to the health of children following IVF is the complications related to prematurity associated with multiple births. Despite the risks associated with multiple pregnancy, couples still tell us every day that they would "love to have twins."

The goal of every treatment cycle should be the delivery of a full-term, healthy, singleton baby.

The ASRM has published guidelines for making the decision of how many embryos to transfer (see Table 4). Patients who fall into the excellent prognosis category should transfer only one or two embryos, whereas those with an exceedingly poor prognosis—because of the woman's age or multiple failed IVFs, for example—may undergo embryo transfer of five or more embryos.

Table 4   Recommended limits on the numbers of embryos to transfer.

Cleavage Stage Embryos[a]			
Prognosis	**Age < 35**	**Age 35–37**	**Age 38–40**	**Age > 40**
Favorable[b]	1–2	2	3	5
All others	2	3	4	5
Blastocysts[a]			
Prognosis	**Age < 35**	**Age 35–37**	**Age 38–40**	**Age > 40**
Favorable[b]	1	2	2	3
All others	2	2	3	3

[a]See text for more complete explanations. Justification for transferring more than the recommended number of embryos should be clearly documented in the patient's medical record.

[b]Favorable = First cycle of IVF, good embryo quality, excess embryos available for cryopreservation, or previous successful IVF cycle.
Source: Adapted from Guidelines on the number of embryos transferred. The Practice Committee of the Society for Assisted Reproductive Technology and the American Society for Reproductive Medicine. *Fertil Steril* 86 [Suppl 4] 2006.

The most problematic decisions concern those patients who fall between these two extremes. Couples who are paying out of pocket for IVF will often pressure their RE to be more aggressive in terms of the number of embryos transferred. Of course, the expense involved in caring for premature infants is many times greater than the cost of all of the fertility procedures used to initiate those pregnancies. The financial costs are merely one part of the picture, as caring for patients with preterm labor or premature infants is also associated with a variety of emotional, psychological, and physical costs.

If multiple pregnancies occur, a multifetal selective reduction procedure can be considered. This procedure is performed at approximately 10 weeks of pregnancy and involves injecting a salt solution into one or more of the gestational sacs. The overall pregnancy loss rate following this procedure is usually less than 5%. In patients who wish to avoid a triplet gestation (but who will not consider selective reduction), it is best to limit the number of embryos transferred to one or two.

Kristin comments:

During my first IVF cycle, we transferred two embryos. This was the standard at our clinic based on my age. When the attempt failed, I was ready to increase the number of embryos transferred to three to increase my chances of getting pregnant. I began another fresh IVF cycle and, when we got close to the transfer, I discussed my desire to transfer three embryos with my RE. He suggested we wait to make the decision based on our embryo quality.

On the day of my transfer, the embryologist refused to transfer more than two embryos because he deemed the two best to be of excellent quality. When I became pregnant with twins, I was extremely thankful that my doctors held their ground and did not let me talk them into transferring more embryos. I had a very difficult pregnancy. If my husband and I decide to try IVF again, we will seriously consider transferring one embryo to reduce my risk of carrying multiples again.

55. How can you have an ectopic pregnancy after IVF?

As described in Part 3, an ectopic pregnancy can occur within the section of the fallopian tube that passes through the muscle of the uterus or within the short segment of fallopian tube that remains after surgical removal of the tube. The incidence of ectopic pregnancy following IVF ranges from 0.5 % to 3%, but this figure may be decreasing. For the past several years, embryo transfer has been routinely performed using ultrasound to properly guide the embryo catheter to the optimal uterine location.

The exact mechanism responsible for an ectopic pregnancy following an IVF procedure is unknown. Some believe that embryo migration up into the fallopian tubes occurs because of local cellular activity or fluid mechanics present inside the uterus. Sometimes the opening of the fallopian tube in the uterus is dilated because of disease, making it easier for the embryos to enter the tubes.

The incidence of an ectopic pregnancy following IVF ranges from 0.5% to 3%.

56. Are there age or other restrictions on who should do IVF?

Age restrictions for IVF vary from clinic to clinic. In general, women older than age 40 have a markedly lower chance for a live birth compared with women younger than 40 years old. Age is probably the most important factor influencing the outcome of an IVF cycle. Many clinics will not treat patients older than age 42, and some malpractice carriers dictate that physicians not perform IVF on patients more than 43 years old with their own eggs because of the poor IVF delivery rates related to advancing age.

A woman's chances for successful IVF can also be predicted by measurement of her FSH and estradiol levels on cycle day 3. Elevations in either hormone are associated with poor IVF success rates, so many clinics impose additional restrictions once the FSH or estradiol levels are known to be elevated. The clomiphene citrate challenge test (CCCT) is another means by which to assess ovarian reserve and predict IVF success. Older women, those with elevated FSH levels on cycle day 3, and those with elevated estradiol levels may consider IVF with donor eggs or adoption.

57. What is ICSI, and how does it differ from IVF?

In routine IVF, eggs are placed in a laboratory dish in culture media together with prepared sperm. The eggs and sperm are allowed to spontaneously fertilize and grow until the embryo transfer procedure, which is usually performed 3 to 5 days after the egg retrieval.

Intracytoplasmic sperm injection (ICSI) differs from IVF in that each egg is individually injected with a single sperm using a tiny needle under microscopic guidance (Figure 4). The resulting embryo is then cultured similarly to an embryo produced in a non-ICSI IVF treatment.

ICSI was initially introduced by the IVF team working at the Brussels Free University in Belgium. At that time, assisted fertilization was being attempted through the insertion of the sperm under the eggshell (**zona pellucida**). The Belgian group took the extra step of injecting the sperm not only under the eggshell but

In ICSI, each egg is individually injected with a single sperm.

Zona pellucida

The outer cellular membrane that surrounds the egg and embryo up to the blastocyst stage of development.

Figure 4 Photograph of an actual ICSI being performed in a laboratory. A holding pipette (A) holds the egg (B) in place. Within the ICSI needle (C), the sperm (D) can be seen. The sperm was injected immediately after this photo was taken. © 2006 American Society for Reproductive Medicine.

actually into the middle of the egg itself. The first ICSI pregnancies were reported in 1992. Since then, tens of thousands of
children have been born as a result of this unique procedure.

Both ICSI and non-ICSI IVF have similar pregnancy rates
and outcomes. The embryos produced by either method
should not be considered to be superior to those created
with the other. ICSI is simply a method to ensure that the
egg is fertilized. ICSI is a safe and proven IVF method that
does not increase the likelihood that the child conceived in
this way will have a birth defect.

58. Who needs ICSI, and how can my repro-
ductive endocrinologist be certain that I need it?

Most couples undergoing treatment with IVF do not require
ICSI. The most common indication for ICSI is male factor
infertility associated with an abnormal semen analysis. For
example, men with unproven fertility whose sperm count,
motility, or morphology is suboptimal may require IVF with
ICSI to ensure fertilization of the ova.

Another common indication for ICSI is unexplained infertility. In these couples, neither the man nor the woman has any
apparent fertility-related problems. Their diagnostic evaluation is entirely normal, yet infertility exists. In such couples,
traditional IVF may result in failure of the man's sperm to
fertilize the woman's eggs. By using ICSI, the eggs are "forced"
to fertilize, and the pregnancy rates are usually high.

59. My husband and I were told by one RE
that we needed ICSI, but another RE says
that we don't. What should we do?

ICSI is accepted as a standard treatment option for infertile
couples with severe male factor infertility. In most clinics,
approximately 50% to 90% of the eggs that are injected
with sperm using ICSI will fertilize normally. Some eggs

do not survive after injection with the sperm and subsequently degenerate.

Approximately 50% to 90% of the eggs that are injected with sperm using ICSI will fertilize normally.

The criteria regarding what constitutes severe male factor infertility, however, vary from clinic to clinic. Some clinics use ICSI for all (or nearly all) patients based on the theory that assisted fertilization is better than no fertilization at all. In general, ICSI is employed in cases where the semen analysis reveals abnormalities related to sperm count (less than 20 million/mL), sperm motility (less than 50% are motile), or sperm morphology (less than 30% have a normal shape). ICSI should also be considered in couples with no previous evidence of fertilization or a history of failed fertilization with a prior IVF attempt.

In our clinic, we often perform an IVF/ICSI split. That is, the eggs that are collected during the oocyte retrieval phase are divided between normal fertilization and ICSI. If some component of male factor infertility is present, splitting the eggs between ICSI and IVF may reveal whether the sperm can actually fertilize an egg. If the eggs fail to fertilize with IVF but fertilize normally with ICSI, then the logical conclusion would be that the sperm is incapable of fertilizing the egg with IVF alone. Couples with unexplained fertilization failure with IVF may have a problem with the sperm, the egg, or both. In such cases a repeat cycle of IVF using ICSI will usually yield good fertilization results and, ideally, a pregnancy.

60. What is the Sperm Chromatin Structure Assay (SCSA), and should my husband have it done?

Sperm Chromatin Structure Assay (SCSA®)

A laboratory test used to determine the degree of DNA fragmentation within a sperm sample.

The **Sperm Chromatin Structure Assay (SCSA)** has been proposed as a means to predict the likelihood of pregnancy in cases of male factor infertility. This test analyzes the degree of DNA fragmentation present in a representative sample of sperm. Increased levels of DNA fragmentation seem to be associated with reduced pregnancy rates, including poorer treatment outcomes with IVF and ICSI. There is no level of fragmentation above which pregnancy is completely ruled out, however, so the SCSA cannot ultimately provide a means to absolutely recommend the use of donor sperm over the sperm from the male partner. If a couple is making a choice between the use of donor sperm compared with partner sperm, then the SCSA may provide a relative indication to use the donor sperm option. At this time, most experts consider this test to be experimental.

61. I was told I need assisted hatching. What is this, and why is it done?

Dr. Gordon's older brother Steven used to tease him by claiming that he was hatched and not born, but actually all of us do "hatch" in early embryonic life. The human embryo hatches out of the eggshell (zona pellucida) at the blastocyst stage of development. **Assisted hatching** involves weakening the zona to facilitate the emergence of the embryo following its transfer into the uterus after IVF. Proponents of assisted hatching suggest that it increases implantation and pregnancy rates.

Assisted hatching

The process of making a small hole in the shell (zona pellucida) surrounding the embryo prior to embryo transfer to promote its implantation in the uterus.

Assisted hatching is almost always performed chemically. In this technique, a dilute acid solution is used to dissolve the external eggshell. Some clinics, however, perform mechanical hatching, in which a slit is made in the eggshell, or even laser-assisted hatching, in which a laser is used to thin the zona. (See Figure 5).

There is some controversy regarding which patients benefit most from assisted hatching, and the indications for assisted hatching remain somewhat unclear. Most clinics recommend this step in cases where the female partner is older than age 37, has diminished ovarian reserve with increased levels of FSH, or is undergoing a frozen embryo transfer (FET) with previously cryopreserved embryos. Patients who have previously failed IVF following replacement of good-quality embryos may also benefit from assisted embryo hatching.

The risks of assisted hatching are believed to be quite low. There have been reports of increased rates of identical twinning following mechanical hatching (but not after chemical-

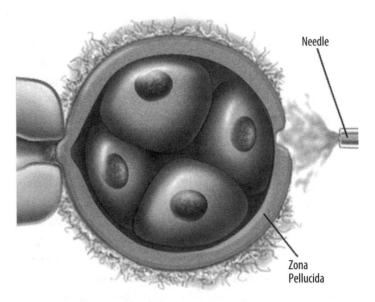

Needle

Zona
Pellucida

Figure 5   Assisted Hatching © 1995 Humanatomy® Illustrated

assisted hatching). There is no evidence that assisted hatching harms the embryo or causes any increased rate of birth defects in children.

Carol comments:

After my first IVF attempt failed for no obvious reason, the RE suggested that we utilize assisted hatching during our second attempt. We immediately moved into a second fresh cycle and employed assisted hatching. From my perspective, there was no difference. The procedure happened after the egg retrieval, so I was not involved. I did get pregnant during the second cycle, and in theory, the assisted hatching was the primary variable that was different.

62. Which types of drug protocols are used in IVF, and how is the most appropriate protocol selected?

Although several drugs and protocols are available to stimulate the ovaries to produce extra eggs for IVF, most clinics utilize only these methods of stimulation. (See Tables 5, 6, and 7 for a list of drugs.)

Table 5   Gonadotropin Preparations

Trade Name, Manufacturer	Source
FSH/LSH-containing preparations	
Pergonal, Serono*	Urine of menopausal women
Repronex, Ferring	Urine of menopausal women
Menopur, Ferring	Urine of menopausal women
Humegon, Organon*	Urine of menopausal women
FSH-containing preparations	
Bravelle, Ferring	Urine of menopausal women
Fertinex, Serono*	Urine of menopausal women
Gonal-F, Serono	Recombinant, Chinese hamster ovary cells
Follistim, Organon	Recombinant, Chinese hamster ovary cells
LH-only-containing preparation	Recombinant
Luveris, Serono	

FSH, follicle-stimulating hormone; LH, luteinizing hormone.
*Drug has been discontinued.

Table 6   Human Chorionic Gonadotropin Preparations

Trade Name, Manufacturer	Source	Formations
Profasi, Serono*	Urine of pregnant females	10,000 IU IM
Pregnyl, Organon	Urine of pregnant females	10,000 IU IM
Novarel, Ferring	Urine of pregnant females	10,000 IU IM
Chorex, Hyrex	Urine of pregnant females	10,000 IU IM
Ovidrel, Serono	Recombinant, Chinese hamster ovary cells	250 μg SC

*Drug has been discontinued.

Table 7   Gonadotropin-Releasing Hormone Agent Agonist/Antagonist Preparations

Trade Name, Manufacturer	Formulations
Lupron Depot, TAP	1 mg/0.2mL = 20 U SC
Synarel, Searle	2 mg/mL intranasal
Zoladex, AstraZeneca	3.6 mg SC
Antagon, Organon	250 μg/0.5 mL SC
Cetrotide, Serono	250 μg/1 mL SC

Luteal suppression

A stimulation protocol that involves suppression of the pituitary gland and ovary prior to initiating stimulation with fertility medications.

Flare stimulation protocol

A technique of follicular stimulation that begins at the start of a spontaneous menstrual cycle.

The first method, called **luteal suppression,** involves suppression of the ovaries using a GnRH-analog (Lupron) during the luteal phase of the menstrual cycle preceding the planned IVF treatment cycle. Once the ovaries are suppressed, ovarian stimulation is accomplished with daily injections of gonadotropins (e.g., Gonal-F, Follistim).

In the second method, called **flare stimulation,** the woman does not take any medications until the second day of her menstrual cycle. At that time, a microdose (most commonly) of Lupron is used to "flare" the pituitary gland and induce it to release its store of FSH and LH. Simultaneously, gonadotropins are started, producing a "one–two punch" in terms of ovarian stimulation. Premature ovulation of the eggs rarely occurs despite the low dose of GnRH agonist utilized in this protocol.

A third, more recent option is GnRH-antagonist stimulation, in which GnRH antagonists are added later in the stimulation to prevent premature ovulation. In this method, the gonadotropins are started on cycle day 2 of a normal menstrual period. Once the follicles have reached a specific size (usually 12 to 14 mm), the woman begins the GnRH-antagonist medication, which almost instantaneously prevents the pituitary gland from generating an LH surge.

Some reproductive endocrinologists prescribe oral contraceptive pills to their female patients prior to beginning the actual ovarian stimulation drugs, but this practice varies between patients and fertility clinics. We have found that the use of birth control pills often results in oversuppression of the ovaries and cycle cancellation except in those patients known to be high responders (women with PCOS, in particular).

The type of protocol selected for any patient (i.e., luteal suppression, flare stimulation or GnRH antagonist) depends on the individual patient and the philosophy of the fertility clinic. Factors that may influence the type of stimulation protocol selected include the patient's age, her day 3 hormone levels, her follicle antral count as determined by ultrasound, and her previous responses to any other attempts at ovarian stimulation.

63. What is natural cycle IVF? And why does my fertility clinic not offer this treatment?

The use of natural-cycle IVF (NC-IVF) has been proposed as a means of reducing the risk of multiple pregnancies, eliminating the costs and risks associated with fertility drugs, and reducing the stress and time commitment needed for traditional stimulated IVF. This approach has been espoused by a number of leaders in the field of IVF, including Dr. Robert Edwards, whose pioneering work along with Dr. Patrick Steptoe's led to the birth of the world's first IVF baby, Louise Brown, in 1978.

"It only takes 1 good egg and 1 good embryo to produce a baby," says Dr. DiMattina.

NC-IVF avoids the use of ovarian stimulation drugs, which cost about $4000 per treatment cycle. With NC-IVF the risks of ovarian hyperstimulation, multiple pregnancy, and the issues of cryopreserved extra embryos are avoided as only one embryo is produced. Total costs are about 20% to 25% of the total cost of conventional IVF.

However, NC-IVF has its own set of disadvantages. For example, by not using fertility drugs, unexpected premature "LH surging" or ovulation can occur, leading to cancellation of the planned egg retrieval. This occurs in about 20% to 30% of treatment cycles. In such cases, if the fallopian tubes are open, the doctor may recommend converting the treatment to an intrauterine insemination (IUI) to try to produce a pregnancy. Furthermore, because only one egg and one embryo are produced, the chances for pregnancy are less than with conventional IVF where two or more embryos are typically replaced. Proponents of NC-IVF expect the "cumulative" pregnancy rate for NC-IVF to be similar to a single cycle of conventional IVF within one to four treatment cycles of NC-IVF.

The best candidates for NC-IVF are patients with regular menstrual cycles who are less than 36 years old and have a normal day three FSH level. Patients with tubal-factor infertility or male factor infertility may be good candidates for NC-IVF before resorting to conventional IVF. Patients with poor ovarian reserve or unexplained infertility will probably experience poorer outcomes with NC-IVF compared with those patients with male factor or tubal factor infertility.

Many European fertility centers routinely use NC-IVF with good success rates. For a variety of reasons, the availability of NC-IVF in the United States has been limited. We believe that NC-IVF will soon become increasingly available as patients demand less stressful and less costly fertility treatments that utilize little to no fertility drugs with good pregnancy rates.

64. My reproductive endocrinologist has recommended a protocol that uses birth control pills. Why would birth control pills be used in IVF?

Birth control pills or, more correctly, oral contraceptive pills (OCPs) can be used as a part of the IVF stimulation protocol in several different settings.

First, in patients who are known or suspected to be high responders, OCPs may help mitigate the risk of ovarian hyperstimulation syndrome (OHSS; see Question 67).

Second, in patients without predictable regular menstrual cycles, OCPs can be used in combination with Lupron to initiate an IVF cycle. In our practice, we usually start OCPs in such cases after confirming with a blood test that the woman has not recently ovulated. Then, after 1 week, we add Lupron. After 1 more week, we stop the Lupron and wait for withdrawal bleeding. Once a patient has bled, we begin the gonadotropin stimulation.

Third, some clinics use OCPs for microdose Lupron (MDL) flare, traditional flare, or patients who are taking Antagon in the hope that pretreatment with OCPs will prevent one follicle from growing faster than the other follicles once the stimulation has begun. We have not routinely use OCPs with our MDL flare patients, as we have rarely had problems with the emergence of a single dominant follicle compared with the more common problem of oversuppression and a cancelled cycle. Given that prolonged OCP use can lead to oversuppression in low responders, we use these medications very carefully.

Prolonged OCP use can lead to oversuppression in low responders.

65. I had an allergic reaction to the progesterone in oil shots. Does this mean that I cannot do IVF?

Following follicle aspiration, most clinics place patients on progesterone supplementation. The rationale behind the supplemental progesterone is that following egg collection, ovarian hormone production may be impaired because many of the hormone-producing cells are removed at the time of follicle aspiration. In addition, the use of GnRH agonists such as Lupron may diminish ovarian steroid production following egg collection. Progesterone supplementation has evolved over the years to include patients undergoing both stimulated IUI cycles and IVF.

Although most clinics tend to use progesterone-in-oil injections, excellent pregnancy rates have been reported in patients who used vaginal progesterone supplementation. Because the progesterone shots are either sesame or peanut oil based, allergic reactions are not infrequent; switching patients to vaginal progesterone preparations usually resolves the problem.

The use of HCG boosters may also increase the woman's risk of ovarian hyperstimulation syndrome.

Another strategy to maintain progesterone production after IUI or egg collection involves the use of HCG booster shots to enhance steroid production from the patient's ovaries rather than relying on an outside source. Unfortunately, the use of HCG boosters may also increase the woman's risk of ovarian hyperstimulation syndrome.

66. My doctor has prescribed estrogen for me but the package says not to take it if you are pregnant. What should I do?

As noted in earlier questions, the ovary produces both estrogen and progesterone until this role is taken over by the placenta at approximately 8 to 10 weeks of pregnancy. Estrogen and progesterone are hormones that are critical for the normal development of the endometrial lining of the uterus. In patients undergoing a frozen embryo transfer (FET) or donor-egg IVF, first estrogen thickens the lining and then progesterone causes the lining to mature, ultimately allowing for the embryo's implantation. Without these hormones, all FET cycles would have to be performed in tandem with natural menstrual cycles and donor-egg IVF would be possible only using frozen embryos, as there would be no way to synchronize the reproductive cycles of the donor and the recipient. There is no evidence that the estrogen used to synchronize these cycles presents any risk to the developing fetus or baby.

If there are no risks, then why do the labels of these medications carry such a strong warning? The labeling is an overreaction to previous experience in the United States with the use of a synthetic estrogen called diethylstilbestrol (DES).

During the 1960s, this synthetic estrogen (which is *not* the natural estrogen used today) was given to women who were threatening to miscarry. Unfortunately, DES did not function in a normal fashion in terms of how it interacted with the estrogen receptors in the cells of the developing female reproductive tract in the unborn daughters of mothers were prescribed DES. As a result, many of those women whose mothers took DES during their pregnancy were found to have significant reproductive tract abnormalities. In addition to cervical and uterine abnormalities, they were at a higher risk for an unusual form of vaginal cancer called clear cell carcinoma. Appropriately, DES was taken off the market. At this point in time, the impact of previous DES exposure in the U.S. population has greatly waned.

Following the DES debacle, the U.S. government decided that all reproductive steroids should be labeled as being contraindicated in pregnancy. This mandate applies to both progesterone and estrogen compounds. Today, however, the estrogens and progesterones prescribed by fertility physicians are exactly equivalent to the body's own natural estrogen and progesterone produced by the ovary and by the placenta. Women who are prescribed these medications by their physician can take them without any worry that somehow these medications will have an adverse impact on their unborn children.

67. My doctor said that I might get ovarian hyperstimulation syndrome. What is ovarian hyperstimulation syndrome, and what can I do to prevent it?

Ovarian hyperstimulation syndrome (OHSS) is a complication associated with the use of fertility drugs. As the ovarian follicles grow, they secrete a wide range of substances, the most important of which is estrogen. Estrogen causes the lining of the uterus to thicken, enabling the embryo to implant there after ovulation and embryo transfer.

Ovarian hyperstimulation syndrome (OHSS) is a complication associated with the use of fertility drugs.

After a woman receives an HCG injection, her follicles eventually collapse, releasing the eggs within; the follicles may also be aspirated with a needle to harvest the eggs for IVF. Within a few days, the fluid within the follicles is restored. Each follicle is now called a corpus luteum (Latin for "yellow body"), referring to the fact that it contains large stores of cholesterol that are used to produce the steroid hormones estrogen and progesterone. In addition, the follicle begins to produce a host of other growth factors—including vascular endothelial growth factor (VEGF), a protein that is likely responsible for the emergence of OHSS.

Mild OHSS results in enlarged, tender ovaries but usually only minimal free fluid in the abdominal cavity. By contrast, moderate and severe forms of OHSS are associated with fluid accumulation in the abdominal cavity or sometimes even in the pleural cavity surrounding the lungs. In its severe form, OHSS can result in nausea, vomiting, shortness of breath, and dehydration. As the fluid builds up in the abdomen, the woman becomes increasingly uncomfortable, and diminished blood flow to the kidneys may lead to decreased urine production. This situation can spiral downward rapidly, and complications of blood clot formation and kidney damage can occur if OHSS is left untreated.

Paracentesis

Placement of a needle through the abdominal wall so as to remove excess abdominal fluid.

Patients with severe OHSS are best managed in the hospital, where they can receive intravenous resuscitation and the fluid can be removed via **paracentesis**. Occasionally, the fluid around the lungs may need to be removed if the woman is suffering from respiratory difficulties. However, most of the respiratory complaints associated with OHSS result from the inability of the diaphragm to move appropriately given the marked amount of fluid present within the abdomen.

Patients with severe OHSS are best managed in the hospital.

Prevention of OHSS is always the best strategy. This syndrome can best be avoided by judicious use of fertility medications, which is why most physicians individualize gonadotropin doses based on the patient's history, the appearance of her ovaries on ultrasound, and her previous response (if any) to fertility medications. Patients older than age 35 in whom fewer than 12 eggs are retrieved rarely develop significant hyperstimulation. In contrast, patients with polycystic ovarian syndrome are at the highest risk for developing OHSS. Other high-risk patients include women who have many small and medium-size follicles associated with estrogen levels of more than 4000 pg/mL at the time of HCG administration. However, not all patients who fall into this category will develop OHSS, and some women who might not otherwise seem to be at risk for it will, in fact, go on to develop the syndrome. This randomness of OHSS makes the decision-making process somewhat problematic when trying to prevent this complication.

A woman who exhibits an excessive response to fertility medications associated with a large number of follicles and a high estrogen level should be counseled regarding OHSS prevention strategies. The first option is to withhold the HCG trigger shot, cancel the cycle, and avoid any attempt at pregnancy. Alternatively, a reduced amount of HCG (5000 units) can be given, followed by follicle aspiration, egg fertilization, and freezing of the embryos with no fresh transfer in that cycle. In such cases, the severe form of hyperstimulation is rarely encountered. In our practice, we have experienced outstanding pregnancy rates during subsequent FET cycles in these patients. Even if no transfer is performed, the woman may still require a brief hospitalization or drainage of the abdominal fluid. Ultimately, it is the HCG trigger shot or the HCG produced by a successful pregnancy cycle that induces the ovarian production of VEGF and the other substances that are the cause of OHSS.

In patients who are stimulated without GnRH agonists (Lupron), an alternative method to reduce the risk of hyperstimulation is to use Lupron itself as a trigger rather than HCG. Given that the majority of women undergoing IVF are already taking Lupron, however, this strategy would apply to only a small percentage of the patients pursuing infertility treatment. Furthermore, this strategy would simply eliminate the initial symptoms of OHSS associated with the HCG trigger shot; if pregnancy subsequently occurs, the patient would still be at risk for the OHSS associated with a successful cycle.

OHSS is an unpleasant experience for patients, but fortunately the incidence of severe OHSS is low (only 1% to 2%) and the vast majority of patients recover quickly with no long-term problems. In cases where OHSS is associated with pregnancy, this problem can last 2 to 3 weeks and may require several procedures to drain the excess fluid. In addition, because of the dehydration associated with OHSS, patients with this syndrome are at risk for the formation of blood clots in the leg or lung. To prevent this complication, most hospitalized patients receive prophylactic daily doses of a blood thinner such as **heparin** or Lovenox.

Heparin
An injectable medication that is used to prevent blood clot formation.

68. Why would my doctor suggest IVF if all of my tests are normal?

Upon completion of the diagnostic evaluation, approximately 10% to 15% of couples will be found to have unexplained infertility, meaning that all of their tests are normal. Such couples are probably best called "subfertile," and most can successfully conceive with IVF. Prior to the introduction of IVF, couples with unexplained infertility had a poor chance of achieving pregnancy with other treatment methods.

We do not know precisely why couples with unexplained infertility are infertile. Some evidence suggests that the source of the problem may be tubal dysfunction or sperm egg interaction. Often, a fertility center uses IVF together with ICSI in such couples to ensure that fertilization of the ova occurs. Thanks to these techniques, today couples with unexplained infertility have a very strong likelihood of ultimately achieving a successful pregnancy with IVF.

Couples with unexplained infertility have a very strong likelihood of ultimately achieving a successful pregnancy with IVF.

69. What is a blastocyst transfer?

Embryos on the third day after egg collection are referred to as cleavage-stage embryos. At this point, each embryo contains 6 to 10 discreet cells (**blastomeres**). When assessing these embryos for quality, the embryologist grades them based on the number and appearance of the blastomeres. Embryos that have equal-size blastomeres with no fragmentation are usually given a high grade, whereas embryos that have extensive fragmentation with unequal-size blastomeres are given a low grade. In general, higher-grade embryos have a much better chance of implanting successfully and generating a pregnancy.

If the embryos are maintained in culture beyond day 3, they first form a solid ball containing approximately 30 to 50 cells, called a **morula**. Over the next day or two, this solid ball of cells becomes a hollow sphere with a clearly defined inner cell mass. This hollow ball of cells is called a blastocyst. Many clinics maintain the embryos in culture until the fifth day to allow for improved selection of embryos to transfer. Patients who undergo an embryo transfer on day 5 or 6 after egg collection are referred to as having a blastocyst transfer. (See Figure 6.)

70. My clinic allows me to choose between a day-3 and a day-5 embryo transfer. How do I decide?

The decision to transfer embryos on day 3 or day 5 is one that requires careful thought. In general, embryos that have formed blastocysts have a better chance of implanting successfully. Unfortunately, not all embryos will progress to the blastocyst stage outside of the body. This inconsistency raises the question as to whether the embryos that fail to form a blastocyst would have initiated pregnancy had they been transferred back into the uterus on day 3. Some studies have, indeed, demonstrated acceptable pregnancy rates with day-3 transfers of embryos

Blastomeres
The individual cells present in an early cleavage-stage embryo.

Morula
An early stage of embryonic development in which the embryo consists of a solid ball of cells; the morula is formed prior to the blastocyst.

Patients who undergo an embryo transfer on day 5 or 6 after egg collection are referred to as having a blastocyst transfer.

4-cell stage

Morula

A mature oocyte undergoing fertilization

Blastocyst (5th day)

Figure 6   Stages of Embryo Development © 1997 Humanatomy® Illustrated

that were of marginal quality and that, based on historical data, would have been unlikely to form blastocysts in culture. Clearly, the pregnancy rate in the absence of an embryo transfer will be zero, whereas even embryos of borderline quality, if transferred on day 3, may potentially lead to a pregnancy.

So how can you decide between a day-3 and a day-5 embryo transfer? Many clinics make the decision on day 3. If a patient has a certain number of high-quality embryos on day 3, then the embryos are maintained in culture for 2 additional days to allow for further embryo selection at the time of transfer. If the embryos fail to progress to the blastocyst stage, however, then there is no transfer—which often results in profound patient disappointment. If a limited number of embryos are available on day 3 and no embryo selection is needed, then the benefit of a day-5 embryo transfer may be limited.

One additional risk of a day-5 transfer is an increased rate of identical twinning. Carrying identical twins (**monozygotic twins**) is considered to be a higher-risk pregnancy than carrying fraternal twins (**dizygotic twins**). Identical twins often share a placenta (**monochorionic twins**) or may even be located within the same pregnancy sac (**monoamniotic twins**); both of these conditions are associated with increased rates of pregnancy complications.

71. My endometrium is only 6 to 7 millimeters thick. Can I do anything to improve its thickness?

The thickness of the endometrium normally changes throughout the menstrual cycle. During menstruation, the endometrium is shed. Under the influence of the hormone estradiol, the endometrium then regenerates and usually develops to a normal thickness of 8 or more millimeters (mm). When a woman is undergoing infertility treatment, the thickness of her endometrium is regularly measured using ultrasonography.

When the endometrium fails to develop to at least 8 mm, the embryo may fail to implant because of endometrial immaturity or dyssynchrony. Although this problem is not very common, when it occurs, it can be difficult to correct. Typical treatments consist of providing additional estrogen early in the menstrual cycle or altering the timing of progesterone administration. Other therapeutic agents include small doses of aspirin (80 to 100 mg per day), and some physicians have prescribed Viagra vaginal suppositories for their female patients with variable success. Some women cannot achieve pregnancy in a fresh IVF embryo transfer cycle but readily become pregnant when the embryos are transferred in a frozen–thawed nonstimulated treatment cycle. On rare occasions, a couple may need to use a gestational carrier to successfully overcome abnormalities involving the endometrium and implantation.

Monozygotic twins

twins arising from a single fertilized egg (also called identical twins).

Dizygotic twins

Twins resulting from the implantation of embryos from two different eggs (also called fraternal twins).

Monochorionic twins

Monozygotic twins who share a single placenta.

Monoamniotic twins

Monochorionic (identical) twins who share a single gestational sac. Carrying monoamniotic twins is considered to be a very high-risk pregnancy.

Preimplantation genetic screening (PGS)

An evaluation that is similar to preimplantation genetic diagnosis but is used to screen embryos in fertility patients for aneuploidy instead of a specific genetic disease.

Autosomal recessive diseases

Genetic diseases carried on a chromosome other than the X or Y chromosomes (sex chromosomes), in which two abnormal copies of the gene are necessary for the disease to be present.

Couples who undergo PGD do not have infertility but rather are at risk for passing a genetic disease to their children; couples who undergo PGS include infertile patients without an underlying genetic problem.

Of course, failure of the endometrium to achieve a minimum thickness of 8 mm does not necessarily translate into a *problem* with the endometrium. In our practice, we have seen many patients with maximal endometrial development of only 4 to 7 mm successfully achieve pregnancy, including delivery of twins. A variety of testing methods to assess endometrial maturity have been proposed, including endometrial biopsy testing for surface proteins called integrins, but such testing is currently considered experimental.

72. What are PGD and PGS?

Preimplantation genetic diagnosis (PGD) and **preimplantation genetic screening (PGS)** are techniques that provide diagnostic information concerning an embryo prior to its transfer to the uterus. The vast majority of PGD and PGS procedures are performed by removing 1 or 2 cells (or blastomeres) of a 6- to 8-cell embryo on day 3 of embryo culture following IVF. These cells are rapidly analyzed, and on day 5 the unaffected embryos are selected for embryo transfer.

PGD was first performed in 1989 in an effort to avoid the transfer of embryos that carried serious genetic disorders (for example, cystic fibrosis). Thus couples who undergo PGD do not have infertility but rather are at risk for passing a genetic disease to their children. A wide range of single-gene and chromosomal disorders can now be diagnosed with PGD, including **autosomal recessive diseases** (e.g., cystic fibrosis), **X-linked recessive diseases** (e.g., hemophilia, Duchenne muscular dystrophy), **autosomal dominant diseases** (e.g., Huntington's disease), and chromosomal rearrangements (e.g., **balanced translocations**).

PGS is similar to PGD, but refers to screening of embryos produced in the course of fertility treatments. Thus couples who undergo PGS include infertile patients without an underlying genetic problem. PGS is performed in an attempt to identify those embryos that are genetically abnormal so that improved embryo selection will—ideally—result in improved pregnancy rates and lower miscarriage rates.

73. How safe is PGD or PGS?

An estimated 5,000 cycles of PGD/PGS are being performed in the United States each year. Although the use of these techniques is clearly increasing, the number of PGD/PGS cycles continues to represent only a small fraction of the 100,000 IVF procedures performed annually in the United States alone. The rate of congenital anomalies and of pregnancy complications following PGD/PGS does not appear to be increased over the baseline measurements.

On occasion, misdiagnosis may occur, so patients undergoing PGD/PGS are usually offered traditional prenatal diagnostic tests (chorionic villus sampling-CVS or amniocentesis) to confirm the results. The rates of misdiagnosis in PGD range from 1% to 9%. Embryos from which no diagnostic information is obtained are usually discarded rather than risk embryo transfer, although this policy varies from clinic to clinic. The other risks of PGS/PGD are the same as those associated with any cycle of IVF, including multiple pregnancy and OHSS.

74. Can PGS improve outcomes after IVF?

PGS has been promoted as a means to improve the odds of a successful IVF cycle. However, a large-scale, randomized, controlled study performed in women older than age 37 failed to demonstrate an improvement in clinical outcome following its use. Although the use of PGS will likely decrease the rate of miscarriage resulting from **aneuploidy** (an abnormal number of chromosomes in the embryo), the overall delivery rate per IVF cycle initiated may not be increased with this technology.

For couples in whom the use of prenatal diagnosis and possible pregnancy termination are not an option, PGS may be appropriate. According to an October 2006 monograph produced by the European Society of Human Reproduction and Embryology (ESHRE), "Although widely used, PGS is

Treatment Options: In Vitro Fertilization

X-linked recessive disease

A genetic disease associated with a mutation on the X chromosome. A male carrying such a mutation will have the disorder because he has only one X chromosome, but a female carrying a mutation on just one X chromosome has a normal gene on the other chromosome and so will not be affected by the disease.

Autosomal dominant diseases

Genetic diseases carried on a chromosome other than the X or Y chromosomes (sex chromosomes), in which a single abnormal copy of the gene leads to the presence of the disease.

Balanced translocation

A chromosomal rearrangement in which two chromosomes break apart and re-form as a new chromosome containing parts of both of the original chromosomes.

still considered as an experimental procedure, and its clinical utility is not fully proven."

One limitation of PGS is that many embryos at the 6- to 8-cell stage of development are mosaics, meaning that some of these cells carry a normal complement of chromosomes while other cells are abnormal. During further embryonic development, the abnormal cells presumably end up relegated to the placenta while the normal cells produce a healthy embryo. The high rate of **mosaicism** in cleavage-stage embryos raises a real concern about the accuracy of PGS. One respected geneticist has estimated a rate of misdiagnosis to be 20% with PGS. Approximately 17% of the time a normal embryo is incorrectly labeled as abnormal and discarded. Even more concerning is the 3% chance that an abnormal embryo will be labeled normal and then transferred to the uterus.

Aneuploidy

Having an abnormal number of chromosomes.

Mosaicism

The presence of both genetically normal and abnormal cells within an embryo prior to implantation.

Many embryos at the 6- to 8-cell stage of development are mosaics—a defect that might potentially escape detection by PGS.

75. What is embryo freezing, and how successful is it?

On the day of embryo transfer, the couple may learn that they have additional embryos of good quality in addition to those embryos that have been selected for embryo transfer. These embryos can be cryopreserved by freezing them in liquid nitrogen. Through a series of carefully orchestrated steps, the embryos are ultimately frozen at a temperature of −196 °C, leaving them in a state of suspended animation in which they can remain for many years. Embryos that have been stored for more than 10 years have successfully generated pregnancies (although most patients tend to use their frozen embryos within 3 to 5 years after they are produced). The pregnancy rates associated with replacing frozen embryos depend on the age of the patient and the quality of the embryos at the time of cryopreservation. Top-quality embryos from young patients may yield pregnancy rates around 50%, whereas poor-quality embryos may not even survive the thawing process. In some clinics, more than 75% of embryos survive the freeze–thaw cycle.

In some clinics, more than 75% of embryos survive the freeze–thaw cycle.

Many couples are often concerned about their moral obligations concerning their frozen embryos. In such cases, couples may elect to defer embryo freezing, choose to alter their stimulation or pursue natural cycle IVF so as to avoid this problem of excess embryos. Extra embryos that are not used to initiate a pregnancy could represent a source of embryonic stem cells. This potential use of extra embryos lies at the heart of the recent political debate in the United States regarding government funding of stem cell research. Clearly, patients should carefully consider the implications of excess frozen embryos as they embark on an IVF cycle. However, not all patients will have extra embryos of high enough quality to be considered for embryo cryopreservation.

76. What is the difference between a natural-cycle frozen embryo transfer (FET) and a medicated FET?

There are two possible options for performing a frozen embryo transfer (FET): natural-cycle FET and medicated FET.

Natural-cycle FET is available to women with regular ovulation and monthly menstrual cycles. In patients with predictable menstrual cycles, we can carefully monitor the cycle to determine the precise timing of ovulation. Alternatively, ovulation can be induced with the administration of an HCG injection. Once the precise date of ovulation is set, then the uterine lining should be receptive to embryo transfer 5 days later (for embryos frozen on day 3 in a previous IVF cycle). In this way, the embryos can be replaced at approximately the time when they would normally be arriving in the uterus.

One problem with natural-cycle FET is that the optimal time for implantation may fall at an unpredictable time during the laboratory work schedule. In addition, natural-cycle FET demands frequent patient monitoring around the time of ovulation. If a cycle is suboptimal in terms of the estrogen level and endometrial development, then the embryos should not be thawed and the cycle should be cancelled.

A medicated FET allows the couple to avoid some of the pitfalls associated with a natural-cycle FET. In this type of FET, estrogen pills, shots, or patches are used to prepare the endometrium for embryo implantation. Three days prior to embryo transfer, the woman begins taking progesterone to modify the endometrial lining so that it will be receptive when the embryos are placed. Some clinics prescribe GnRH agonists (such as Lupron) to their female patients the month prior to a medicated FET cycle so as to reduce the chances of spontaneous ovulation. The use of Lupron reduces the chances of cycle cancellation owing to unexpected ovulation to near zero.

The choice of estrogen supplementation varies somewhat between clinics. Some clinics prescribe oral estrogens, other clinics administer intramuscular estrogen shots twice a week, and still other clinics ask their patients to use transdermal estrogen patches twice a week. The choice of estrogen protocol is clinic-specific and should be discussed with your reproductive endocrinologist.

Most clinics prescribe progesterone-in-oil injections to prepare the lining for embryo transfer. Women who have a progesterone allergy can use progesterone suppositories or Prometrium capsules, instead.

Pregnancy rates have not been shown to differ significantly between natural-cycle FET and medicated FET. However, medicated FETs do allow for advance scheduling, which both patients and physicians find attractive.

77. My last IVF failed. Should I try again?

To make the best decision about whether to do another IVF, your first step is usually to sit down with your doctor and re-

> *A medicated FET allows the couple to avoid some of the pitfalls associated with a natural-cycle FET.*

view your history and the details of the failed cycle. This would include a discussion of the rationale behind attempting IVF in the first place and a careful examination of the results of the IVF cycle. Clearly, if a woman can conceive only through the use of IVF (for example, because she has no fallopian tubes or because her partner's sperm is of such poor quality that no other alternative is available), then the decision becomes one of whether another attempted IVF is warranted.

In reviewing the previous IVF cycle, the woman's response to the stimulation protocol should be carefully examined as well as the findings at the time of egg collection. If the eggs appeared immature at the time of egg collection, then in the future the trigger shot should probably be withheld until the follicles reach a larger diameter. If the stimulation and number of eggs are appropriate but fertilization was unexpectedly poor, then the use of ICSI for a future IVF cycle could be considered. If stimulation, fertilization, and embryo development were good and yet the cycle still failed, then consideration should be given to either an FET cycle (if appropriate) or a repeat cycle of IVF. If the stimulation was poor and the number of eggs was suboptimal, then other stimulation protocols should be discussed. If maximum doses were used and a poor response was still seen, then IVF may not be an appropriate choice; in such a case, other options—ranging from IUI to donor egg or adoption—may warrant discussion.

In cases where patients have frozen embryos remaining from the fresh IVF, we usually encourage them to attempt pregnancy with a frozen embryo transfer. Many patients who fail to conceive on a fresh IVF will conceive on the FET.

Many patients who fail to conceive on a fresh IVF will conceive on the FET.

The post-IVF consultation is one of the most useful discussions that a couple can have with the physician. It allows the couple to review all aspects of their care and to determine whether IVF represents the best approach to their particular situation. We firmly believe that this feedback is crucial to develop an appropriate plan of treatment for each couple.

Kristin comments:

Obviously, this is a very personal decision that is based on your own emotional, physical, and financial situation. For us, the answer was easy: Yes! At our post-cycle consult with the RE, he reassured us that IVF could work for us. We discussed the quality of our remaining frozen embryos and the chances of conceiving through a FET and ultimately decided to pursue another fresh IVF cycle. We jumped right back into IVF, doing two back-to-back fresh cycles. They were not easy months, emotionally or physically. I had wonderful support from family and friends, and this helped to keep me focused on my ultimate goal of creating a family with my husband. I believe it is very important to have somebody to discuss your fears, concerns, and frustrations with while cycling, be it an online buddy, family member, friend, or professional counselor. So often the focus is on the financial and physical ramifications of IVF, but the emotional toll is often the worst.

78. When can I do a home pregnancy test after IVF?

Hormonal detection of pregnancy may be performed by testing for the presence of the hormone beta-HCG in either the urine or the blood. Both types of tests are reliable and highly accurate. Sometimes, however, a home urine pregnancy test can be misleading and give a spuriously negative or positive test result when performed too early (regardless whether the desired pregnancy is from an IVF treatment or a spontaneous conception). Performing a pregnancy test within 7 days after the egg collection procedure can result in a false-positive result because of residual HCG after the shot is given to trigger the final maturation of the eggs. In addition, the urine pregnancy test may be spuriously negative if performed less than 14 days after the embryo transfer. In our practice, we have had patients with a serum beta-HCG level of more than 200 mIU/mL who nevertheless had a negative urine pregnancy test.

We advise patients to obtain a blood pregnancy test 12 to 14 days after an IVF embryo transfer and to avoid home pregnancy testing. In-office blood pregnancy tests provide the most reliable and accurate result.

Kristin comments:

Our RE highly encouraged us to wait for the blood test, and my husband was extremely adamant that I not do a home pregnancy test. He did not want me to be given false hope by a positive home pregnancy test that turned out not to be a viable pregnancy. The 2-week wait was extremely difficult, but we kept ourselves busy by planning a 5-day trip in the middle of it.

I am really glad I did not do a home pregnancy test with our first IVF because it probably would have been positive, despite the outcome of a chemical pregnancy. To have the hope of pregnancy erased the next day by a low beta would have been more than I could handle emotionally at the time. On our second IVF attempt I waited until I got the positive beta from the RE, and then I took many home pregnancy tests so I could see that double line for myself.

We advise patients to obtain a blood pregnancy test 12 to 14 days after an IVF embryo transfer and to avoid home pregnancy testing.

79. When I went in for my first ultrasound after IVF, my RE saw two gestational sacs at 6.5 weeks, but only one had a fetal pole with a heartbeat. What will happen to the other pregnancy sac?

Such events are not uncommon following IVF. The incidence of a clinical twin pregnancy after IVF is 10% to 25%, with the exact likelihood depending on the number of embryos transferred and the age of the patient. In 30% to 40% of these pregnancies, one gestational sac will be empty, a situation called a blighted ovum pregnancy. Often, these pregnancies will simply disappear. At other times, the woman may experience cramping and bleeding. In such a case, there is a 40% to 50% risk that the healthy gestational sac and fetus will also abort. There is no way to predict the outcome, and there is no medical intervention that can be implemented to preserve the normal sac and fetus. During this difficult time, patients are well advised to rest and decrease their stress as much as possible. Supplemental progesterone may help quiet uterine contractions, but it is not curative.

In women who suffer a twin early pregnancy loss, a medical investigation may be indicated to search for any organic causes that may have contributed to the early pregnancy loss. Unfortunately, such evaluations usually do not produce any definitive answers.

Carol comments:

During my first pregnancy, I lost a twin at 8 weeks after fetal cardiac activity was visualized. I do recall a severe episode of cramping, but there was no bleeding involved. In addition to my RE, the other medical professionals involved confirmed that no intervention was necessary. I went on to enjoy a very normal pregnancy and delivered my son at 40.5 weeks.

80. My beta-HCG levels are as follows: 260 mIU/mL 14 days after a day-3 embryo transfer, 500 mIU/mL 16 days post transfer, 900 mIU/mL 18 days post transfer, and 1900 mIU/mL 20 days post transfer. Is there any hope for this pregnancy?

In a normal early pregnancy, regardless of the method of conception, the woman's blood beta-HCG levels will roughly double every 48 hours. Failure of the beta-HCG levels to double suggests an abnormal intrauterine pregnancy or an ectopic pregnancy. Given that biologic variation can occur in both normal and abnormal pregnancies, however, we cannot assume that a pregnancy is in jeopardy simply because the beta-HCG levels fail to perfectly double.

In the case described in the question, the woman's beta-HCG levels did not double, but she could have either a normal in-

Failure of the beta-HCG levels to double suggests an abnormal intrauterine pregnancy or an ectopic pregnancy.

trauterine pregnancy, an abnormal intrauterine pregnancy, or an ectopic pregnancy. This determination can be made only by performing a transvaginal ultrasound examination. Even then, the results may be inconclusive. In our practice, we have seen several cases in which patients had dramatically abnormal beta-HCG levels associated with a first sonogram, suggesting an early blighted ovum pregnancy, only to discover later that the pregnancy was completely normal.

Another common cause for abnormal increases in the beta-HCG level is multiple pregnancy. When patients undergo transfer of two or more embryos, a multiple gestational pregnancy may occur. In roughly 40% of these pregnancies, spontaneous fetal reduction of the extra implanted sacs occurs, resulting in a sudden drop in the beta-HCG level. Initially this decrease might be falsely interpreted as an apparent problem with the pregnancy when, in fact, one surviving embryo is completely healthy. For all these reasons, the blood beta-HCG doubling effect must be viewed as a guide, and not as absolute proof of the woman's condition and future outcome of her pregnancy.

PART NINE

Treatment Options: Third-Party Reproduction

Why does my reproductive endocrinologist think that I need to use an egg donor?

What are egg donors, and how is donor egg–IVF performed?

Where do egg donors come from, and why do they want to be a donor?

More . . .

81. Why does my reproductive endocrinologist think that I need to use an egg donor?

A woman is born with all of her eggs and is incapable of making more over the course of her lifetime. After the age of 30, her fertility begins to decline—markedly so after the age of 35. By age 40, most women will experience infertility.

Egg quality can be assessed, to a limited degree, by obtaining blood hormone levels for FSH and estradiol on cycle day 3. Elevations in either hormone suggest diminishing ovarian reserve. Another test for ovarian reserve is the clomiphene citrate challenge test (CCCT), a simple blood test that measures FSH and estradiol before and after the woman takes Clomid. Many reproductive endocrinologists perform an ovarian transvaginal ultrasound examination and a follicle count to further assess ovarian function. Often, the blood FSH, estradiol, and follicle counts are normal, yet the woman fails to respond to treatment. Thus normal hormone levels can be misleading—but abnormal levels usually suggest that an egg-related problem truly exists.

When a woman's eggs fail to respond adequately to treatment, when the woman has failed to conceive with previous attempts at IVF or other treatments, or when she has abnormal ovarian reserve, then IVF using donor eggs is an excellent option. Since 1984, egg donation has been a cornerstone in treating patients whose eggs have deteriorated either through the normal aging process or because of disease. By using donated eggs from a woman in her twenties, the infertile patient essentially restores her fertility potential to that of her egg donor. Similarly, the miscarriage rate drops from more than 50% for patients older than age 40 to 10% to 12% with the use of donor eggs.

Egg donation has been used extensively in patients who are **perimenopausal** or even menopausal. Most clinics enforce an age restriction in terms of their egg-donor recipients, with

Since 1984, egg donation has been a cornerstone in treating patients whose eggs have deteriorated either through the normal aging process or because of disease.

Perimenopause

The years preceding the last menstrual cycle characterized by increasingly irregular cycles, hot flashes, and low estrogen levels.

the most common cut-off age being 50 years old. Unlike the eggs, the uterus slowly ages and remains receptive to implantation (as long as the endometrium is successfully prepared with hormones) well into a woman's fifth and possibly sixth decades of life.

82. What are egg donors, and how is donor egg–IVF performed?

Donor egg–IVF involves the use of healthy female egg donors who are usually in their twenties. Most donor arrangements are anonymous, although known donor egg IVF is possible. In the latter case, the known donors are usually family members or friends. In our experience, most of our patients prefer to use an anonymous egg donor to avoid family and interpersonal conflicts.

Most medical practices recruit egg donors for their patients, but third-party agencies are also available that act as brokers. The American Society of Reproductive Medicine (ASRM) has developed a set of egg-donor screening guidelines, which most practices utilize for screening donors. The guidelines encompass comprehensive screening for infectious and genetic diseases, physical examination, and psychological testing. Since May 2005, the U.S. Food and Drug Administration (FDA) has mandated extensive infectious disease testing in screening all anonymous egg and sperm donors.

The actual treatment cycle for donor-egg IVF essentially combines a fresh IVF cycle (the donor) and a medicated FET cycle (the recipient). The two treatment cycles are synchronized by using GnRH analogs. Usually, the recipient begins estrogen therapy 5 days prior to the start of the egg donor's stimulation so as to provide an adequate time frame for the recipient's endometrium to grow and thicken. After 10 to 14 days of stimulation, the donor receives an injection of HCG (Pregnyl, Profasi, Ovidrel) to mature her eggs. On the same day, the recipient starts progesterone therapy to create a receptive endometrium.

Because most egg donors are young, they tend to respond very well to the ovarian stimulation drugs, producing many high-quality eggs and embryos. Implantation rates with these embryos are also very high, so that usually only one or two embryos are transferred to the recipient. Pregnancy rates usually exceed 50% per initiated cycle, making donor-egg IVF the most successful therapy currently available for infertile couples. Usually, extra embryos that were not transferred can be frozen and stored for later transfer, with excellent pregnancy rates achieved in subsequent conception attempts.

Pregnancy rates usually exceed 50% per initiated cycle of donor-egg IVF.

83. Where do egg donors come from, and why do they want to be a donor?

The typical egg donor is a healthy, young female in her twenties who desires to help others in having a baby. In our experience, egg donors tend to be intelligent, altruistic, sincere women who are knowledgeable about the difficulties that many couples face with their infertility. Most egg donors come from the local community near the infertility practice. They have learned about infertility from their friends, family, the Internet, and the media.

Most of the donors whom we recruit for our practice have a college degree or are actively pursuing one. Most anonymous donors are reimbursed for their time and the expenses involved in the screening and treatment process. The screening usually takes 2 to 3 months to complete and the IVF treatment takes 4 to 6 weeks.

In our experience, women who donate their eggs are very responsible individuals and genuinely concerned about carefully completing their role in the IVF treatment process to achieve a successful outcome.

84. What screening tests are performed on donors?

Both the ASRM and the FDA have issued clear screening guidelines and regulations for egg and sperm donors;

the guidelines are available on these organizations' respective websites. A typical evaluation involves a comprehensive history of the donor's health and his or her family. A physical examination and comprehensive laboratory screening tests for communicable diseases are also performed. Many centers add genetic testing of the donors. A psychological assessment of all ova donors is routinely performed.

Although the anonymous donor's anonymity is preserved, the results of his or her laboratory tests, psychological profile, physical characteristics, and historical information are shared with the infertile couple. This information allows couples to carefully choose their donor and provides a certain level of comfort in knowing that proper screening was performed. Some clinics provide adult photos of their donors, but in our practice we have limited photos to those from childhood to preserve the donors' anonymity.

85. What is a gestational carrier, and when should you consider using one?

Fertility doctors sometimes recommend the use of a third-party gestational carrier if the infertile couple wants to have their own biological child. Many medical conditions necessitate the use of a gestational carrier, including the absence of a uterus in the would-be mother, either because of a congenital (at birth) condition or when a disease necessitated its surgical removal. A gestational carrier may also be the best option when a woman has a systemic disease that may affect either her own or her baby's health, such as advanced heart disease, severe diabetes, or multiple sclerosis. Likewise, a woman with a history of poor pregnancy outcome—including repetitive pregnancy losses, preterm labor, **incompetent cervix,** or severe **preeclampsia**—may be a good candidate for IVF using a gestational carrier.

Prior to the IVF treatment, thorough screening of the gestational carrier is routinely performed using ASRM guidelines. Gestational carriers are usually well known to the couple and

Incompetent cervix

A muscular-fibrous weakening of the cervix, leading to painless cervical dilation and second-trimester or early third-trimester pregnancy loss.

Preeclampsia

A vascular disease of pregnancy characterized by hypertension, edema, and a risk of seizure.

may be relatives or friends. In addition, agencies exist that introduce gestational carriers to prospective patients. In such arrangements, the gestational carrier is usually compensated for her time and energy (especially if the pregnancy proves successful).

When using a gestational carrier, IVF is performed by combining the infertile couple's sperm and eggs to produce their own genetic embryos. However, unlike in standard IVF, these embryos are then transferred into the uterus of the gestational carrier. This process resembles donor-egg IVF in that the process requires synchronization of two patients: the egg donor (genetic parent) and the recipient (gestational carrier). Pregnancy proceeds normally just as if the gestational carrier had become spontaneously pregnant. The major factor in determining the success rate is the age of the woman whose eggs are donated. The ideal gestational carrier is a woman who has had a previous uncomplicated pregnancy and delivery.

The ideal gestational carrier is a woman who has had a previous uncomplicated pregnancy and delivery.

PART TEN

Stress, Exercise, and Alternative Medications

What role does stress play in causing infertility?

Can I exercise? How much is okay?

One of my friends tried acupuncture before her IVF cycle and it worked! Should I try acupuncture?

More . . .

86. What role does stress play in causing infertility?

Not surprisingly, dealing with infertility can itself be very stressful. And stress—both physical and psychological—can significantly affect a woman's ability to conceive. A recent study examining the role of psychological stress in successful pregnancy showed a one-third decrease in pregnancy rates in those women undergoing IVF who perceived themselves to be overly stressed. Most of these women were lawyers whose stress was perceived to be job related.

Excessive physical stress can also be detrimental to a woman's ability to conceive. Studies show that women who run more than 20 miles per week may begin to experience abnormalities in their menstrual cycle, which may in turn affect their fertility potential. Women who run marathons or compete at a very high physical level, for example, commonly have ovulatory dysfunction and infertility.

Excessive physical stress can also be detrimental to a woman's ability to conceive.

There are many different ways to decrease the stress inherently present with infertility and its treatment—for example, decreasing work hours or changing jobs, exercise, meditation, yoga, acupuncture, getting a new hobby, or simply setting aside some time for oneself. Many patients are able to reduce their infertility-related stress by simply becoming more knowledgeable about the subject of infertility. In addition to providing physician counseling, we ask our own patients to read and become more educated about their infertility, thereby empowering them to take control of it. Excellent and reliable information is available at the American Society of Reproductive Medicine website (www.ASRM.org).

Carol comments:

Looking back on my experience, I do think that my level of stress and daily environment played a major role in my inability to conceive naturally. When I did a fresh cycle to get pregnant the second time, I had been out of the corporate environment for over a year. Not only was the quality of my embryos better, but I was able to achieve a successful pregnancy during the first fresh cycle. Obviously, it's not possible for everyone to leave their job for an extended period while attempting to get pregnant, but I do agree that anything that can be done to reduce stress is a positive contribution.

87. Can I exercise? How much is okay?

Mild to moderate exercise is beneficial to infertility patients and is highly encouraged. Healthy amounts of exercise decrease stress and clearly improve a person's sense of well-being. Studies show that women who exercise before and during their pregnancy have better obstetrical outcomes and healthier babies than women who are sedentary. For most patients, we recommend exercising 30 minutes per day, 4 or 5 times per week, but lesser amounts of exercise are still beneficial. Even 15 minutes of exercise each day can help reduce stress and improve your physical health.

We highly recommend that women begin or continue exercising during their infertility evaluation and treatments, and perhaps more so for those undergoing treatment with IVF. In our experience, these patients are better able to tolerate the stress related to infertility and IVF.

88. One of my friends tried acupuncture before her IVF cycle and it worked! Should I try acupuncture?

It is unclear whether acupuncture really improves the IVF pregnancy rates. Several studies have suggested an improvement in IVF pregnancy rates with acupuncture. In addition, acupuncture may help in decreasing the stress of infertility, which may in turn indirectly improve the likelihood for success with IVF. Decreasing stress during the infertility treatment process is always a good thing. The excellent work of Alice

Domar, PhD (Domar Center for Complementary Healthcare, Waltham, MA) and others has demonstrated the efficacy of the mind-body approach in relieving distress.

Kristin comments:

I looked into acupuncture during my first IVF cycle. The acupuncturist suggested that I try Reiki, a Japanese form of spiritual healing, because he preferred to treat IVF patients prior to the cycle ever starting. I can't say that Reiki got me pregnant, but it certainly helped me to relax, and that can never hurt. For women experiencing infertility, being told to "just relax" is one of the most insulting things you can hear, but if you can find a stress-reducing activity—be it yoga, massage, Reiki, acupuncture, or even meditating—it can help you to make it through the emotionally draining times.

89. Does being overweight have any effect on infertility or on IVF success rate?

Many studies show that being overweight adversely affects a woman's fertility potential and increases the likelihood for early pregnancy loss and obstetrical complications. Many obese women have irregular or absent menstrual cycles. For many of these individuals, weight reduction alone will restore their normal ovulation and menstrual cycles and enhance their fertility potential. Often, these individuals will spontaneously conceive with no medical therapy once they have reduced their weight.

Body mass index (BMI)

A mathematical calculation that uses height and weight to determine whether an individual is of normal weight, overweight, or obese.

Prior to performing IVF, we discuss with our patients the impact of obesity on their IVF success rates at great length. Most are very appreciative of our concern and advice, and they are generally motivated to reduce their weight so that they will have a greater chance for success with IVF and for an uncomplicated pregnancy. We recommend that obese patients, defined as those with a **body mass index (BMI)** greater than 29), reduce their weight prior to establishing pregnancy.

Sometimes it takes 2 to 6 months of weight reduction to reach the goal prior to the planned IVF treatment. Regardless of the type of infertility treatment planned, weight loss can have a dramatic effect in terms of enhancing the chance of a successful pregnancy.

Fad or crash diets are not recommended when a woman is trying to lose weight prior to infertility treatment, as these practices can be harmful to anyone's general health. Local community nutritionists, organizations such as Weight Watchers, personal physicians, and information available on the Internet such as the American College of Obstetricians and Gynecologists (www.ACOG.org) website can assist in establishing a plan for weight reduction.

90. Does smoking cause infertility?

Smoking significantly harms the fertility potential for both men and women. Women who smoke are at greater risk for experiencing premature menopause (known as premature ovarian failure). Smoking directly affects their egg quality, resulting in increased rates of infertility. In IVF patients, smoking has been shown to dramatically lower the chances for a successful treatment. In addition, the chances for a spontaneous abortion are also increased in smokers compared with nonsmoking women. Smoking also directly affects sperm quality, diminishing both sperm count and sperm motility.

91. Can I drink caffeine and alcohol during my infertility treatments?

Consumption of limited amounts of caffeine and alcohol appears to be safe when attempting to conceive. Drinking 1 to 2 cups of coffee per day, or similar amounts of caffeinated beverages, does not decrease a woman's chances for getting pregnant either naturally or with any of the infertility treatments available. Although several studies suggested that drinking 1 or 2 beers or glasses of wine per day, or the equivalent, also has no adverse effect on fertility, newer information casts

Smoking significantly harms the fertility potential for both men and women.

some doubt upon that view. Unfortunately, there are many confounding variables in this type of research; thus, we suggest that you ask your physician for his/her recommendations.

No amount of alcohol can be considered safe in pregnancy.

Once pregnancy occurs, limited caffeine consumption may continue without any untoward effects to the fetus. By contrast, a woman should avoid consuming even very small amounts of alcohol as soon as pregnancy occurs. Routine use of alcohol can lead to a well-described condition called fetal alcohol syndrome. At this time, the consensus is that no amount of alcohol can be considered safe in pregnancy.

PART ELEVEN

Pregnancy Loss

How common is miscarriage?

What can cause recurrent pregnancy loss,
and can it be treated?

What are the genetic causes of pregnancy loss,
and can they be treated?

More . . .

92. How common is miscarriage?

Human reproduction is extraordinarily inefficient. Pregnancy loss rates are remarkably high at all ages, with 10% to 15% of all clinically recognized pregnancies undergoing spontaneous abortion even in women during their peak fertility years (between 20 and 30 years old). The rates of miscarriage are age related: In women older than age 40, for example, pregnancy loss is greater than 50%.

Many pregnancies are lost so early in development that no gestational sac is ever visualized on sonogram. This type of pregnancy loss is called a biochemical pregnancy. In most cases, once fetal cardiac activity is visualized on ultrasound, the miscarriage rate drops to less than 5%. In women older than age 40, however, the pregnancy loss rate remains 25% or greater even after visualization of cardiac activity. A pregnancy that stops developing in the absence of any bleeding is also called a missed abortion. Remember that the medical term "abortion" refers to any pregnancy loss, either spontaneous or induced. Miscarriage is a lay term that is used to refer to a spontaneous abortion. Although most pregnancy losses occur during the first trimester, adverse outcomes can occur at any gestational age.

Miscarriage is a lay term that is used to refer to a spontaneous abortion.

93. What can cause recurrent pregnancy loss, and can it be treated?

Given that pregnancy loss is a relatively common phenomenon, some patients might suffer several losses without any underlying predisposing factors. However, patients who suffer two or three consecutive spontaneous abortions may benefit from an evaluation to rule out any additional risk factors for poor pregnancy outcome and to determine whether any treatment might potentially reduce the risk of a recurrent loss.

Patients who suffer two or three consecutive spontaneous abortions may benefit from an evaluation.

In general, the causes of recurrent pregnancy loss can be divided into genetic, hormonal, anatomic, infectious, autoimmune, and thrombophilic categories. Approximately 40%

to 50% of patients with two or three consecutive pregnancy losses will be determined to have an apparent etiology (source of the problem). In these cases, treatment would depend on the specific problem identified. In those patients without any obvious etiology of their recurrent pregnancy loss, treatment options include empiric progesterone, empiric baby aspirin, treatment with fertility medications and IUI, IVF, and IVF with preimplantation genetic diagnosis (PGD). Older patients with recurrent pregnancy loss or those with diminished ovarian reserve are probably best treated through the use of donor-egg IVF.

94. What are the genetic causes of pregnancy loss, and can they be treated?

The most common etiology of pregnancy loss is genetic. Sixty to seventy percent of first-trimester pregnancy losses are genetically not normal. The most common class of abnormality is autosomal **trisomies**. In such pregnancies, one extra chromosome is present in the developing pregnancy, causing it to fail. Not all trisomies are lethal, however. For example, trisomy 21 (also known as Down syndrome) can result in a live birth, and children with Down syndrome are fairly well recognized by the population at large. However, most trisomy pregnancies undergo spontaneous miscarriage.

Couples who have suffered two or three consecutive losses are recommended to have their blood tested for **karyotype** analysis to ensure that they are genetically normal. Certain chromosomal rearrangements in the parents can predispose to pregnancies possessing abnormal chromosome arrangements, leading to an increased rate of pregnancy loss or fetal abnormalities. The most common of these parental chromosomal rearrangements is a balanced translocation, in which two different chromosomes (for example, chromosomes 14 and 21) break and exchange genetic information. This rearrangement may lead to unbalanced chromosomal arrangements in the egg or the sperm, subsequently predisposing the pregnancy to

Trisomy

An abnormal genetic condition that arises when an individual possesses three copies of a particular chromosome instead of the normal two copies.

The most common class of genetic abnormality in pregnancy loss is autosomal trisomies.

Karyotype

The chromosomal complement of an individual, including the number of chromosomes and any chromosomal abnormalities.

miscarriage. Although patients with balanced translocations may successfully conceive and deliver healthy babies without assistance, many consider fertility treatments up to and including IVF with preimplantation genetic diagnosis (PGD) to reduce the risk of pregnancy loss.

95. Which hormonal problems can lead to miscarriage?

Several hormonal sources for pregnancy loss have been suggested, including untreated thyroid disease, diabetes, polycystic ovarian syndrome (PCOS), and luteal-phase defects.

Thyroid disease is easily diagnosed through blood tests for thyroid-stimulating hormone (TSH) and thyroid hormone itself (free T_4). Fortunately, thyroid dysfunction responds promptly to treatment.

Although uncontrolled diabetes may lead to an increased risk of pregnancy loss, individuals with this degree of glucose intolerance usually have been identified prior to the pregnancy.

Women with PCOS may experience an increased risk of first-trimester pregnancy loss. It is estimated that these individuals have a 25% chance of first-trimester pregnancy loss compared with a rate of 10% to 15% in an age-matched control group. The mechanism through which PCOS may increase the chance of pregnancy loss is unknown, but limited preliminary studies suggest that the use of metformin (Glucophage) may reverse this tendency.

Women with PCOS have a 25% chance of first-trimester pregnancy loss.

Finally, women who produce a suboptimal amount of progesterone, both in the luteal phase and in early pregnancy, are at increased risk for pregnancy loss. However, testing for such luteal-phase defects remains somewhat problematic and controversial. In our practice, we routinely supplement all patients in the first trimester of pregnancy with progesterone suppositories, obviating the need for additional diagnostic tests such as an endometrial biopsy.

96. Can fibroids or other uterine problems cause miscarriage?

Anatomical abnormalities can predispose a woman to pregnancy loss. In particular, congenital uterine abnormalities such as a uterine septum (fibrous band separating the uterine cavity into two smaller cavities) or a unicornuate uterus (a small malformed uterus that is usually connected to a single fallopian tube) can lead to poor reproductive outcomes. Uterine malformations as a result of prenatal exposure to diethylstilbestrol (DES; see Question 66) can also increase a woman's risk of a poor pregnancy outcome. The presence of uterine fibroids within or abutting the endometrial cavity has been proposed as a source of pregnancy loss (see Figure 7); the same is true of uterine polyps. Extensive **intrauterine adhesions** from a previous dilatation and curettage (D&C) procedure may also lead to reduced reproductive success. All of these abnormalities may be amenable to surgical correction, but the decision to pursue surgery requires a careful discussion with your physician.

Intrauterine adhesions

fibrous bands of tissue found within the uterine cavity.

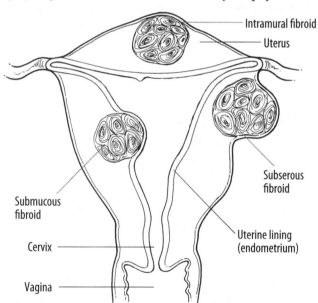

Subserous fibroids are located in the outer wall of the uterus. Intramural fibroids are found in the muscular layers of the uterine wall, and submucous fibroids are located under the uterine lining and protrude into the uterine cavity.

Figure 7   Fibroids © 2006 American Society for Reproductive Medicine.

97. Can an infection cause miscarriage?

Both bacterial and viral infectious sources for recurrent pregnancy loss have been proposed. In particular, the presence of either of two types of bacteria—ureaplasma or mycoplasma—within the cervix or uterus has been suggested as a risk factor for pregnancy loss. The scientific evidence is somewhat lacking to prove this connection, but we routinely culture our patients for ureaplasma and mycoplasma and treat both members of a sexually intimate couple when and if these bacteria are found. Women who become infected with *Listeria* (a type of bacterial food poisoning) after eating unpasteurized dairy products can also miscarry as a result.

Similarly, certain viral infections can cause miscarriage if contracted during pregnancy. **Parvovirus B19** causes a mild viral illness in children known as **fifth's disease**. Children who contract this illness have a fever and bright red cheeks, lending the disease its other common name of "slapped cheek syndrome." Unfortunately, women who contract this illness during pregnancy can suffer miscarriage even in the second and third trimesters. Once infected, an individual becomes immune to this virus, so parvovirus B19 would not cause repetitive pregnancy loss. No vaccine exists for parvovirus B19.

98. Should I have autoimmune tests done if I have a history of miscarriage?

Autoimmune sources of recurrent pregnancy loss should be evaluated, especially in women with a history of rheumatologic or autoimmune disease. Women with a preexisting autoimmune disease such **systemic lupus erythematosus (lupus)** are clearly at risk for pregnancy loss and poor reproductive outcomes. In particular, lupus patients who have **antiphospholipid antibodies** (especially **anticardiolipin antibodies**) are at the highest risk for pregnancy loss. The presence of these antibodies in the absence of lupus also suggests that the woman has an increased risk of miscarriage and poor

Parvovirus B19

A virus that can cause an intrauterine infection leading to fetal anemia, fetal heart failure, and miscarriage.

Fifth's disease

An infectious disease caused by parvovirus B19. It leads to bright rosy checks in children but can cause miscarriage if a woman contracts it during pregnancy.

Systemic lupus erythematosus (lupus)

A systemic auto-immune disease that causes inflammation, arthritis, rash, and other medical problems, including pregnancy loss.

Antiphospholipid antibodies

The general class of antibodies that are formed against various components of the cells of the body; their presence is often associated with pregnancy loss.

pregnancy outcome. Treatment recommendations in such cases include daily pediatric doses of aspirin (81 mg/day), low-dose injectable blood thinners (such as heparin or Lovenox), or both.

Testing for antiphospholipid antibodies in all women who have infertility problems, even if they do not have a history of pregnancy loss, is unwarranted. In our practice, we usually restrict such testing to those patients with a history of pregnancy loss. Women who have a history of pregnancy loss should undergo both antiphospholipid antibodies and lupus anticoagulant testing.

99. What is thrombophilia, and how does it relate to miscarriage?

Over the last several years, there has been an increased interest in evaluating patients with recurrent pregnancy loss for the presence of **thrombophilia**. Thrombophilia literally means "thrombosis-loving"; a thrombosis is a blood clot. All humans exist in a balance between bleeding and blood clotting. Genetic conditions such as hemophilia leave affected individuals open to complications arising from excessive bleeding. Similarly, people who have genetic predispositions to blood clotting can be at risk for problems ranging from blood clots in the lung (pulmonary embolus) or leg (deep vein thrombosis), to an increased risk of miscarriage or poor pregnancy outcomes, including intrauterine fetal demise and intrauterine growth retardation.

Typical tests for thrombophilia include assessment of **Factor V Leiden, prothrombin II, proteins C and S, antithrombin III,** and the **methyltetrahydrofolate reductase (MTHFR)** enzyme. All of these except MTHFR are genetic enzyme deficiencies that cause the affected person to have a propensity toward blood clot formation; these conditions are often treated with pediatric aspirin and heparin (usually Lovenox).

Anticardiolipin antibodies

Specific antibodies that are formed against various components of the cells of the body; their presence is often associated with pregnancy loss.

Women who have a history of pregnancy loss should undergo both antiphospholipid antibodies and lupus anticoagulant testing.

Thrombophilia

A disorder of the blood clotting system resulting in a tendency to form blood clots. It may also lead to a higher risk of miscarriage.

Factor V Leiden

A genetic disorder that predisposes a woman to blood clot formation and miscarriage.

Prothrombin II

A protein involved in the blood clotting system.

Proteins C and S

Proteins involved in the blood clotting system.

Antithrombin III

A protein involved in the coagulation cascade. A deficiency in antithrombin III is associated with an increased risk of blood clotting and pregnancy loss.

Methyltetra-hydrofolate reductase (MTHFR)

An enzyme involved in folic acid metabolism.

People with a MTHFR mutation may be at higher rate for blood clot formation (and miscarriage, if female) if they also have elevated levels of homocystine, a metabolic by-product of folic acid metabolism. People who are positive for two copies of an MTHFR enzyme mutation are best treated with vitamin supplementation consisting of folic acid, vitamin B_6, and vitamin B_{12}. Several preparations have been specifically formulated for these individuals (Foltx or Folgard). Women with thrombophilia are probably best evaluated by a hematologist to review the potential need for anticoagulation before, during, and following any pregnancy.

100. Where can I go to find more information?

Appendix A lists some recommended resources for finding out more about infertility. In addition, Appendix B contains more questions and answers from the CDC's 2004 report on **assisted reproductive technologies (ART)**.

Women with thrombophilia are probably best evaluated by a hematologist to review the potential need for anti-coagulation before, during, and following any pregnancy.

Assisted reproductive technologies (ART)

A variety of fertility procedures (including in vitro fertilization) that involve manipulating sperm and eggs to achieve pregnancy.

Patient Support Groups

The American Fertility Association

The American Fertility Association is a national non-profit organization dedicated to educating, supporting, and advocating for women and men facing decisions related to family building and reproductive health, including prevention and medical treatment of infertility, social and psychological concerns, coping mechanisms, and adoption. The AFA offers many services including publications, seminars, referrals, online educational sessions, coaching support groups, and professionally moderated message boards.
666 Fifth Avenue Suite 278
New York, NY 10103
888-917-3777 (Support Line)
www.theafa.org

The Endometriosis Association

The Endometriosis Association was the first organization in the world created for those with endometriosis. As an independent self-help organization of women with endometriosis, doctors, and others interested in the disease, it is a recognized authority in its field. Its goal is to work toward finding a cure for the disease as well as providing education, support, and research.
8585 N. 76th Place,
Milwaukee, Wisconsin 53223
(For a free packet of information call 1-800-992-3636.)
Tel: 414-355-2200
Fax: 414-355-6065
www.endometriosisassn.org

Fertile Hope

Fertile Hope is a national, nonprofit organization dedicated to providing reproductive information, support, and hope to cancer patients and survivors. Through programs of awareness, education, financial assistance, research, and support, Fertile Hope is helping cancer survivors fulfill their parenthood dreams.
Fertile Hope
PO. Box 624
New York, NY 10014
1-888-994-HOPE
www.fertilehope.org

InterNational Council on Infertility Information Dissemination (INCIID)

The InterNational Council on Infertility Information Dissemination (INCIID—pronounced "inside") is a nonprofit organization that helps individuals and couples explore their family building options. INCIID provides current information and immediate support regarding the diagnosis, treatment, and prevention of infertility and pregnancy loss. It also offers guidance to those considering adoption or childfree lifestyles. Dr. Gordon moderates the IVF and High Tech Pregnancy Bulletin Board on the website.

PO Box 6836
Arlington, VA 22206
703-379-9178
www.inciid.org

International Premature Ovarian Failure Association (IPOFA)

The International Premature Ovarian Failure Association, Inc. (IPOFA) is a nonprofit organization whose mission is to provide community, support, and information to women with Premature Ovarian Failure (POF) and their loved ones, to increase public awareness and understanding of POF, and to work with health care professionals to better understand this condition.

IPOFA
PO Box 23643
Alexandria, VA 22304
703-913-4787 (Support Line)
www.pofsupport.org

Polycystic Ovarian Syndrome Association

The Polycystic Ovarian Syndrome Association exists to provide comprehensive information, support, and advocacy for women and girls with the condition known as polycystic ovary syndrome.

PO Box 3403
Englewood, CO 80111
www.pcosupport.org

RESOLVE: The National Infertility Association

RESOLVE is a nonprofit organization mandated to promote reproductive health and to ensure equal access to all family building options for men and women experiencing infertility or other reproductive disorders. It also provides support services and physician referral and education. The mission of RESOLVE is to provide timely, compassionate support and information to people who are experiencing infertility and to increase awareness of infertility issues through public education and advocacy.

7910 Woodmont Ave, Suite 1350
Bethesda, MD 20814
301-652-6611 (Main Number)
301-652-9375 (Fax)
1-888-623-0744 (Helpline)
www.resolve.org

Professional Organizations

American Society for Reproductive Medicine (ASRM)

American Society for Reproductive Medicine, a nonprofit organization of physicians, nurses, and other healthcare professionals is dedicated to helping patients overcome infertility. The society accomplishes its mission through the pursuit of excellence in education and research, and through advocacy on behalf of patients, physicians, and affiliated healthcare providers.
1209 Montgomery Highway
Birmingham, AL 35216-2809
205-978-5000
www.asrm.org

Society for Reproductive Endocrinology and Infertility

Membership in the Society for Reproductive Endocrinology and Infertility (SREI) is limited to Board Certified Reproductive Endocrinologists. The members of the SREI are dedicated to providing excellence in Reproductive Health through research, education, and the care of their patients. Patients can find the reproductive endocrinologists that practice in their area by clicking on the Find Members link and can obtain additional information by viewing the pdf file for SREI physicians located at the society's website.
www.socrei.org

CDC's Assisted Reproductive Technology Page

Information is available from the CDC on reproductive health sciences. They offer statistics from infertility clinics as well as a multitude of other information pertaining to reproduction.
www.cdc.gov/ART/ART2004/index.htm

Pharmaceutical Industry

Ferring Pharmaceuticals

According to the Ferring Pharmaceuticals website:
When it comes to infertility treatment, look to the leader in science. . . . Our scientists are dedicated to finding innovative solutions to help couples fulfill the dream of

childbirth. Not surprisingly, we are taking the lead in Assisted Reproductive Technology (ART). In fact, Ferring products are the fastest growing fertility brands on the market today.

The information provided at FerringFertility.com has been developed to help patients learn more about infertility as they continue on their journey toward parenthood. This information is not meant to replace communications between healthcare professionals and patients. Healthcare professionals are the best source of medical information for patients. Ferring provides educational materials, videos, and other free information about their products to patients and providers.

Ferring manufactures Bravelle, Menopur, and Novarel.

Ferring Pharmaceuticals Inc.

400 Rella Boulevard, Suite 300

Suffern, NY 10901

1-888-FERRING (Customer Service Line)

www.ferringfertility.com

Organon

According to the Organon website, "Organon is committed to supporting both physicians and patients with proven fertility products for use in assisted reproduction techniques."

Organon sponsors a website that provides more information about fertility and fertility treatment in general: Fertility Journey (http://www.fertilityjourney.com). Fertility Journey is an online resource for patients that provides information, guidance, and support as they undergo fertility treatments. Topics include: testing and diagnosis, therapy options, and coping techniques. In addition, an online clinic locator assists with finding a local IVF clinic for patients in the US. Organon manufactures Follistim and Pregnyl.

Organon USA Inc.

56 Livingston Ave.

Roseland, NJ 07068

1-800-241-8812

http://www.fertilityjourney.com

Serono

According to the Serono website, "Serono is dedicated to providing patient-friendly products and services to help people build families."

In response to the needs of fertility patients, Serono launched Fertility LifeLines, a free and confidential educational service that offers customized information and support to people with fertility health concerns.

Serono manufactures Gonal-F, Ovidrel, and Luveris.

1-866- LETS-TRY (1-866-538-7879)

www.fertilitylifelines.com

SECTION I: OVERVIEW

Where are U.S. ART clinics located, how many ART cycles did they perform in 2004, and how many infants were born?

Although ART clinics are located throughout the United States, generally in or near major cities, the greatest number of clinics is in the eastern United States. Figure 1 shows the locations of the 411 reporting clinics. The fertility clinic section of this report, arranged in alphabetical order by state, city, and clinic name, provides specific information on each of these clinics. The number of clinics, cycles performed, live-birth deliveries, and infants born as a result of ART all have increased steadily since CDC began collecting this information in 1995 (see Section 5, pages 57–68). Because in some cases more than one infant is born during a live-birth delivery (e.g., twins), the total number of infants born is greater than the number of live-birth deliveries. CDC estimates that ART accounts for slightly more than 1% of total U.S. births.

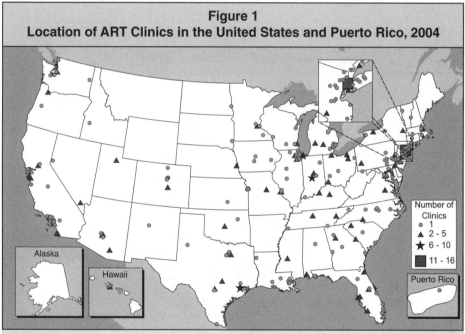

Figure 1
Location of ART Clinics in the United States and Puerto Rico, 2004

Number of
Clinics
○ 1
▲ 2 - 5
★ 6 - 10
■ 11 - 16

Alaska

Hawaii

Puerto Rico

Number of ART clinics in the United States in 2004:	461
Number of U.S. ART clinics that submitted data in 2004:	411
Number of ART cycles reported in 2004:	127,977*
Number of live-birth deliveries resulting from ART cycles started in 2004:	36,760
Number of infants born as a result of ART cycles carried out in 2004:	49,458

*Note: This number does not include 239 cycles in which a new treatment procedure was being evaluated (see Figure 2).

What types of ART cycles were used in the United States in 2004?

For 74% of ART cycles carried out in 2004, fresh nondonor eggs or embryos were used. ART cycles that used frozen nondonor embryos were the next most common type, accounting for approximately 15% of the total. In about 12% of cycles, eggs or embryos were donated by another woman. A very small number of cycles (less than 1% of the ART cycles carried out in 2004) involved the evaluation of a new treatment procedure. The vast majority of these cycles included pre-implantation genetic diagnosis for screening of genetic disorders, and a few involved the retrieval of immature oocytes. The number of cycles in which a new treatment procedure was being evaluated is not included in the total number of cycles reported in Sections 2 through 5 of the national report and in the individual fertility clinic tables. Thus, data presented in subsequent figures in this report and in the individual fertility clinic tables are based on 127,977 ART cycles.

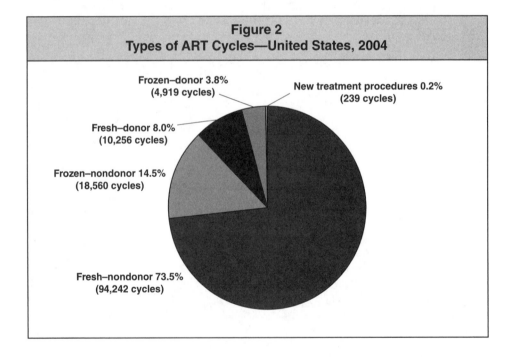

Figure 2
Types of ART Cycles—United States, 2004

Frozen–donor 3.8%
(4,919 cycles)

New treatment procedures 0.2%
(239 cycles)

Fresh–donor 8.0%
(10,256 cycles)

Frozen–nondonor 14.5%
(18,560 cycles)

Fresh–nondonor 73.5%
(94,242 cycles)

How old were the women who used ART in the United States in 2004?

The average age of women using ART services in 2004 was 36. The largest group of women using ART services were women younger than 35, representing 41% of all ART cycles carried out in 2004. Twenty-one percent of ART cycles were carried out among women aged 35–37, 19% among women aged 38–40, 9% among women aged 41–42, and 9% among women older than 42.

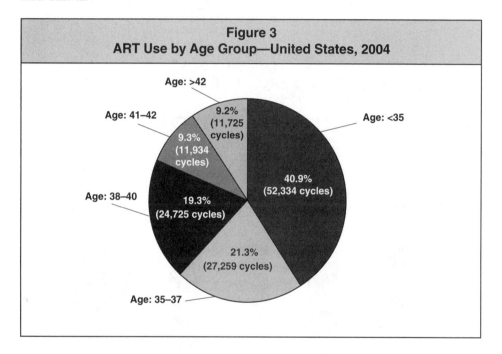

Figure 3
ART Use by Age Group—United States, 2004

- Age: >42 — 9.2% (11,725 cycles)
- Age: 41–42 — 9.3% (11,934 cycles)
- Age: <35 — 40.9% (52,334 cycles)
- Age: 38–40 — 19.3% (24,725 cycles)
- Age: 35–37 — 21.3% (27,259 cycles)

Did the types of ART cycles used in the United States in 2004 differ among women of different ages?

Figure 4 shows that, in 2004, the type of ART cycles varied by the woman's age. The vast majority (96%) of women younger than 35 used their own eggs while only 4% used donor eggs. In contrast, 21% of women aged 41 to 42 and more than half (54%) of women older than 42 used donor eggs. Across all age groups, more ART cycles using fresh eggs or embyos were performed than cycles using frozen embryos.

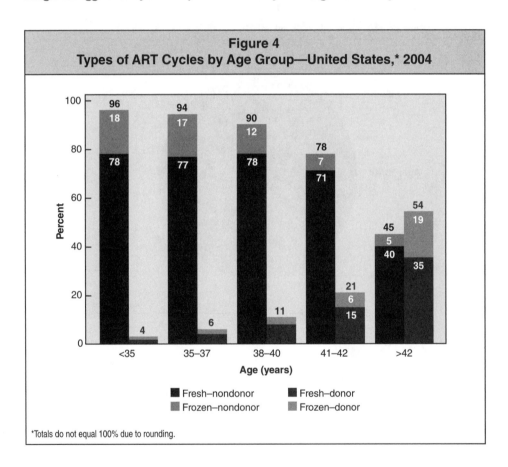

**Figure 4
Types of ART Cycles by Age Group—United States,* 2004**

*Totals do not equal 100% due to rounding.

SECTION 2: ART CYCLES USING FRESH NONDONOR EGGS OR EMBRYOS

What are the steps for an ART cycle using fresh nondonor eggs or embryos?

Figure 5 presents the steps for an ART cycle using fresh nondonor eggs or embryos and shows how ART users in 2004 progressed through these stages toward pregnancy and live birth.

An ART **cycle is started** when a woman begins taking medication to stimulate the ovaries to develop eggs or, if no drugs are given, when the woman begins having her ovaries monitored (using ultrasound or blood tests) for natural egg production.

If eggs are produced, the cycle then progresses to **egg retrieval**, a surgical procedure in which eggs are collected from a woman's ovaries.

Once retrieved, eggs are combined with sperm in the laboratory. If fertilization is successful, one or more of the resulting embryos are selected for **transfer**, most often into a woman's uterus through the cervix (IVF), but sometimes into the fallopian tubes (e.g., GIFT, ZIFT; see pages 504 and 505 for definitions).

If one or more of the transferred embryos implant within the woman's uterus, the cycle then may progress to clinical **pregnancy**.

Finally, the pregnancy may progress to a **live birth**, the delivery of one or more live-born infants. (The birth of twins, triplets, or more is counted as one live birth.)

A cycle may be discontinued at any step for specific medical reasons (e.g., no eggs are produced, the embryo transfer was not successful) or by patient choice.

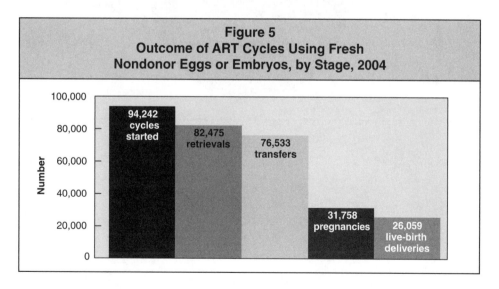

**Figure 5
Outcome of ART Cycles Using Fresh
Nondonor Eggs or Embryos, by Stage, 2004**

Why are some ART cycles discontinued?

In 2004, 11,767 ART cycles (about 12%) were discontinued before the egg retrieval step (see Figure 5). Figure 6 shows reasons that the cycles were stopped. For approximately 83% of these cycles, there was no or inadequate egg production. Other reasons included too high a response to ovarian stimulation medications (i.e., potential for ovarian hyperstimulation syndrome), concurrent medical illness, or a patient's personal reasons.

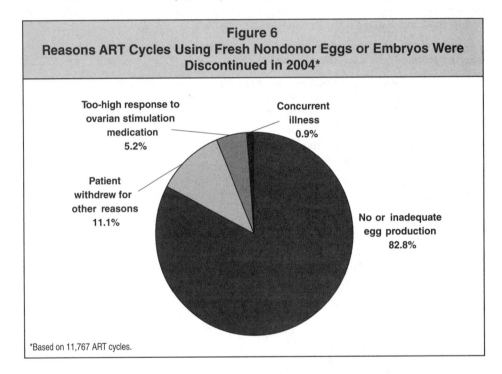

Figure 6
Reasons ART Cycles Using Fresh Nondonor Eggs or Embryos Were Discontinued in 2004*

Too-high response to ovarian stimulation medication 5.2%

Concurrent illness 0.9%

Patient withdrew for other reasons 11.1%

No or inadequate egg production 82.8%

*Based on 11,767 ART cycles.

How is the success of ART measured?

Figure 7 shows ART success rates using six different measures, each providing slightly different information about this complex process. The vast majority of rates have increased slightly each year since CDC began monitoring them in 1995 (see Section 5, pages 57–68).

- **Pregnancy per cycle rate:** the percentage of ART cycles started that produced a pregnancy. This rate is higher than the live birth per cycle rate because some pregnancies end in miscarriage, induced abortion, or stillbirth (see Figure 9, page 21).

- **Live birth per cycle rate:** the percentage of ART cycles started that resulted in a live birth (a delivery of one or more live-born infants). This rate is the one many people are most interested in because it represents the average chances of having a live-born infant by using ART. **Throughout this report, live birth rate means live birth per cycle rate unless otherwise specified.**

- **Live birth per egg retrieval rate:** the percentage of ART cycles in which eggs were retrieved that resulted in a live birth. It is generally higher than the live birth per cycle rate because it excludes cycles that were canceled before eggs were retrieved. In 2004, about 12% of all cycles using fresh nondonor eggs or embryos were canceled for a variety of reasons (see Figure 6).

- **Live birth per transfer rate:** includes only those ART cycles in which an embryo or egg and sperm were transferred back to the woman. This rate is the highest of these six measures of ART success.

- **Singleton live birth per cycle rate:** the percentage of ART cycles started that resulted in a singleton live birth. Overall, singleton live births have a much lower risk than multiple-infant births for adverse infant health outcomes, including prematurity, low birth weight, disability, and death.

- **Singleton live birth per transfer rate:** the percentage of ART cycles that resulted in a singleton live birth among ART cycles in which an embryo or egg and sperm were transferred back to the woman.

Figure 7
Success Rates for ART Cycles Using Fresh
Nondonor Eggs or Embryos, by Different Measures, 2004

What percentage of ART cycles results in a pregnancy?

Figure 8 shows the results of ART cycles in 2004 that used fresh nondonor eggs or embryos. Most of these cycles (66%) did not produce a pregnancy; a very small proportion (0.7%) resulted in an ectopic pregnancy (the embryo implanted outside the uterus), and slightly less than 34% resulted in clinical pregnancy. Clinical pregnancies can be further subdivided as follows:

- 20.3% resulted in a single-fetus pregnancy.

- 11.3% resulted in a multiple-fetus pregnancy.

- 2.1% ended in miscarriage before the number of fetuses could be accurately determined.

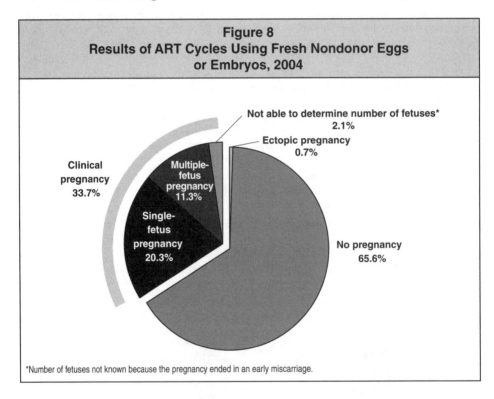

Figure 8
Results of ART Cycles Using Fresh Nondonor Eggs or Embryos, 2004

Not able to determine number of fetuses*
2.1%

Ectopic pregnancy
0.7%

Clinical pregnancy
33.7%

Multiple-fetus pregnancy
11.3%

Single-fetus pregnancy
20.3%

No pregnancy
65.6%

*Number of fetuses not known because the pregnancy ended in an early miscarriage.

What percentage of pregnancies results in a live birth?

Figure 9 shows the outcomes of pregnancies resulting from ART cycles in 2004 (see Figure 8). Approximately 82% of the pregnancies resulted in a live birth (55% in a singleton birth and 27% in a multiple-infant birth). Seventeen percent of pregnancies resulted in an adverse outcome (miscarriage, induced abortion, or stillbirth). For 0.9% of pregnancies, the outcome was not reported.

Although the birth of more than one infant is counted as one live birth, multiple-infant births are presented here as a separate category because they often are associated with problems for both mothers and infants. Infant deaths and birth defects are not included as adverse outcomes because the available information for these outcomes is incomplete.

Figure 9
Outcomes of Pregnancies Resulting from ART Cycles Using Fresh Nondonor Eggs or Embryos, 2004

Using ART, what is the risk of having a multiple-fetus pregnancy or multiple-infant live birth?

Multiple-infant births are associated with greater problems for both mothers and infants, including higher rates of caesarean section, prematurity, low birth weight, and infant disability or death.

Part A of Figure 10 shows that among the 31,758 pregnancies that resulted from ART cycles using fresh nondonor eggs or embryos, 60% were singleton pregnancies, 29% were twins, and about 5% were triplets or more. Six percent of pregnancies ended in miscarriage in which the number of fetuses could not be accurately determined. Therefore, the percentage of pregnancies with more than one fetus might have been higher than what was reported (about 34%).

In 2004, 5,393 pregnancies resulting from ART cycles ended in either miscarriage, stillbirth, or induced abortion, and 299 pregnancy outcomes were not reported. The remaining 26,059 pregnancies resulted in live births. Part B of Figure 10 shows that approximately 33% of these live births produced more than one infant (30% twins and approximately 3% triplets or more). This compares with a multiple-infant birth rate of slightly more than 3% in the general U.S. population.

Although the total rates for multiples were similar between pregnancies and live births, there were more triplet (or more) pregnancies than births. Triplet (or more) pregnancies may be reduced to twins or singletons by the time of birth. This can happen naturally (e.g., fetal death), or a woman and her doctor may decide to reduce the number of fetuses using a procedure called multifetal pregnancy reduction. Information on medical multifetal pregnancy reductions is incomplete and therefore is not provided here.

Figure 10
Risk of Having Multiple-Fetus Pregnancy and Multiple-Infant Live Birth from ART Cycles Using Fresh Nondonor Eggs or Embryos, 2004

Total multiple-fetus pregnancies: 33.5%

Triplets or more 4.9%

Triplets or more 2.6%

Not able to determine number of fetuses* 6.2%

Total multiple-infant live births: 32.5%

Twins 28.6%

Twins 29.9%

Singletons 60.3%

Singletons 67.5%

A. 31,758 Pregnancies

B. 26,059 Live births

*Number of fetuses not known because the pregnancy ended in an early miscarriage.

What are the ages of women who use ART?

Figure 11 presents ART cycles using fresh nondonor eggs or embryos according to the age of the woman who had the procedure. About 12% of these cycles were among women younger than age 30, 68% were among women aged 30–39, and 20% were among women aged 40 and older.

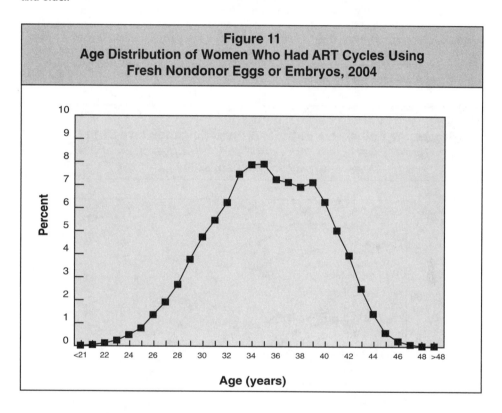

Figure 11
Age Distribution of Women Who Had ART Cycles Using Fresh Nondonor Eggs or Embryos, 2004

Do ART success rates differ among women of different ages?

A woman's age is the most important factor affecting the chances of a live birth when her own eggs are used. Figure 12 shows the pregnancy rates, live birth rates, and singleton live birth rates for women of different ages who had ART procedures using fresh nondonor eggs or embryos in 2004. Live birth rates and singleton live birth rates are different because of the high percentage of multiple-birth deliveries counted among the total live births. The percentage of multiple births is particularly high among women younger than 35 (see Figure 31). Among women in their 20s, pregnancy rates, live birth rates, and singleton live birth rates were relatively stable; however, success rates declined steadily from the mid-30s onward as fertility declined with age. For additional detail on success rates among women aged 40 years or older, see Figure 13.

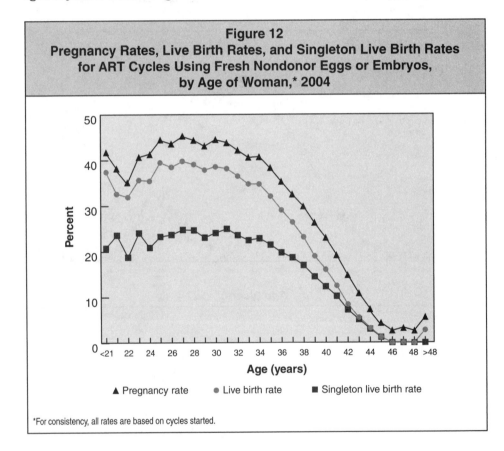

Figure 12
Pregnancy Rates, Live Birth Rates, and Singleton Live Birth Rates for ART Cycles Using Fresh Nondonor Eggs or Embryos, by Age of Woman,* 2004

▲ Pregnancy rate   ● Live birth rate   ■ Singleton live birth rate

*For consistency, all rates are based on cycles started.

How do ART success rates differ for women who are 40 or older?

Success rates decline with each year of age and are particularly low for women 40 or older. Figure 13 shows pregnancy rates, live birth rates, and singleton live birth rates for women 40 or older who used fresh nondonor eggs or embryos. The average chance for pregnancy was 23% for women age 40; the live birth rate for this age was about 16%, and the singleton live birth rate was 12%. All rates dropped steadily with each 1-year increase in age. For women older than 44, the live birth rates and singleton live birth rates were both a little less than 1%. Women 40 or older generally have much higher success rates using donor eggs (see Figure 41, page 53).

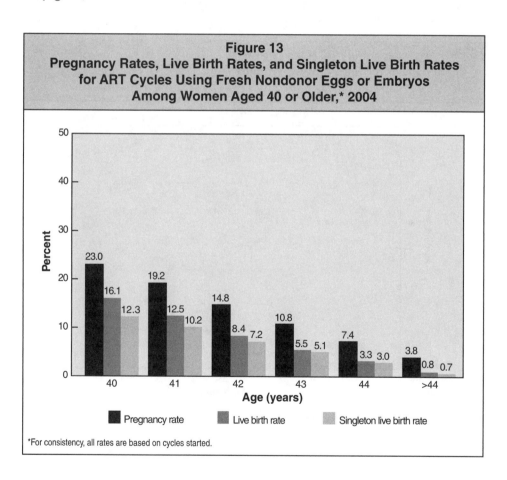

Figure 13
Pregnancy Rates, Live Birth Rates, and Singleton Live Birth Rates for ART Cycles Using Fresh Nondonor Eggs or Embryos Among Women Aged 40 or Older,* 2004

*For consistency, all rates are based on cycles started.

How do miscarriage rates for ART patients vary among women of different ages?

A woman's age not only affects the chance for pregnancy when her own eggs are used, but also affects her risk for miscarriage. Figure 14 shows miscarriage rates for women of different ages who became pregnant using ART procedures in 2004. Miscarriage rates were below 12% among women younger than 34. The rates began to increase among women in their mid- to late 30s and continued to increase with age, reaching 28% at age 40 and 59% among women older than 43.

The miscarriage rates observed among women undergoing ART procedures using fresh nondonor eggs or embryos appear to be similar to those reported in various studies of other pregnant women in the United States.

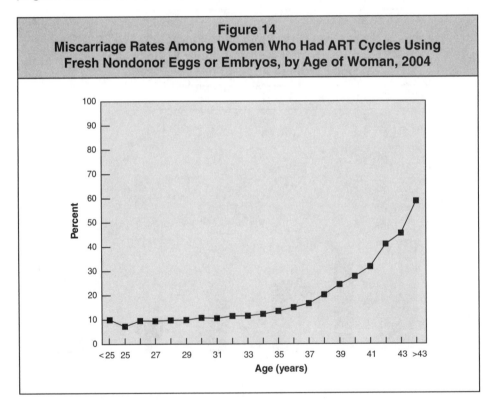

Figure 14
Miscarriage Rates Among Women Who Had ART Cycles Using Fresh Nondonor Eggs or Embryos, by Age of Woman, 2004

How does a woman's age affect her chances of progressing through the various stages of ART?

In 2004, a total of 94,242 cycles using fresh nondonor eggs or embryos were started:

- 40,853 in women younger than 35
- 21,019 in women 35–37
- 19,174 in women 38–40
- 8,487 in women 41–42
- 4,709 in women older than 42

Figure 15 shows that a woman's chance of progressing from the beginning of ART to pregnancy and live birth (using her own eggs) decreases at every stage of ART as her age increases.

- As women get older, the likelihood of a successful response to ovarian stimulation and progression to **egg retrieval** decreases.
- As women get older, cycles that have progressed to egg retrieval are slightly less likely to reach **transfer**.
- The percentage of cycles that progress from transfer to **pregnancy** also decreases as women get older.
- As women get older, cycles that have progressed to pregnancy are less likely to result in a **live birth** because the risk for miscarriage is greater (see Figure 14).

Overall, 37% of cycles started in 2004 among women younger than 35 resulted in live births. This percentage decreased to 29% among women 35–37 years of age, 20% among women 38–40, 11% among women 41–42, and 4% among women older than 42. As noted in Figures 12 and 13, the proportion of cycles that resulted in singleton live births is even lower for each age group.

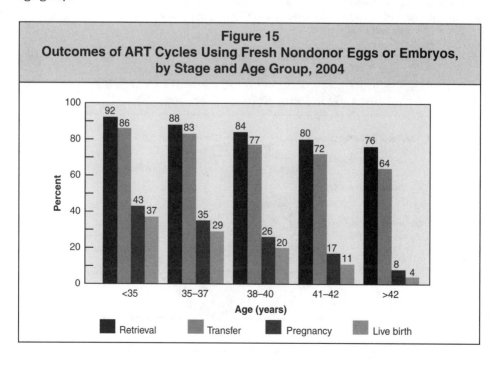

Figure 15
Outcomes of ART Cycles Using Fresh Nondonor Eggs or Embryos, by Stage and Age Group, 2004

What are the causes of infertility among couples who use ART?

Figure 16 shows the infertility diagnoses reported among couples who had an ART procedure using fresh nondonor eggs or embryos in 2004. Diagnoses range from one infertility factor in one partner to multiple factors in either one or both partners. However, diagnostic procedures may vary from one clinic to another, so the categorization may also vary.

- **Tubal factor** means that the woman's fallopian tubes are blocked or damaged, making it difficult for the egg to be fertilized or for an embryo to travel to the uterus.
- **Ovulatory dysfunction** means that the ovaries are not producing eggs normally. Such dysfunctions include polycystic ovary syndrome and multiple ovarian cysts.
- **Diminished ovarian reserve** means that the ability of the ovary to produce eggs is reduced. Reasons include congenital, medical, or surgical causes or advanced age.
- **Endometriosis** involves the presence of tissue similar to the uterine lining in abnormal locations. This condition can affect both fertilization of the egg and embryo implantation.
- **Uterine factor** means a structural or functional disorder of the uterus that results in reduced fertility.
- **Male factor** refers to a low sperm count or problems with sperm function that make it difficult for a sperm to fertilize an egg under normal conditions.
- **Other causes** of infertility include immunological problems, chromosomal abnormalities, cancer chemotherapy, and serious illnesses.
- **Unexplained cause** means that no cause of infertility was found in either the woman or the man.
- **Multiple factors, female only,** means that more than one female cause was diagnosed.
- **Multiple factors, female and male,** means that one or more female causes and male factor infertility were diagnosed.

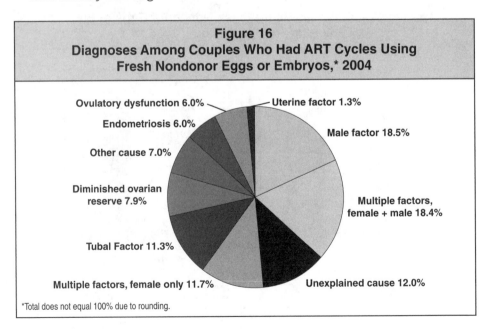

Figure 16
Diagnoses Among Couples Who Had ART Cycles Using Fresh Nondonor Eggs or Embryos,* 2004

Ovulatory dysfunction 6.0%
Uterine factor 1.3%
Endometriosis 6.0%
Male factor 18.5%
Other cause 7.0%
Diminished ovarian reserve 7.9%
Multiple factors, female + male 18.4%
Tubal Factor 11.3%
Multiple factors, female only 11.7%
Unexplained cause 12.0%

*Total does not equal 100% due to rounding.

Does the cause of infertility affect the chances of success using ART?

Figure 17 shows the percentage of live births per ART cycle according to the causes of infertility. (See Figure 16 or the Glossary in Appendix B for an explanation of the diagnoses.) Although the national average success rate was about 28% (see Figure 7), success rates varied somewhat depending on diagnosis; however, the definitions of these diagnoses may vary from clinic to clinic. In general, couples diagnosed with tubal factor, ovulatory dysfunction, endometriosis, male factor, or unexplained infertility had above-average success rates. The lowest success rate was observed for those with diminished ovarian reserve. Additionally, couples with uterine factor, "other" causes, or multiple infertility factors had below-average success rates. Please note, however, that review of select clinical records revealed that reporting of infertility causes may be incomplete. Therefore, differences in success rates by causes of infertility should be interpreted with caution. (See Findings from Validation Visits for 2004 ART Data for additional information.)

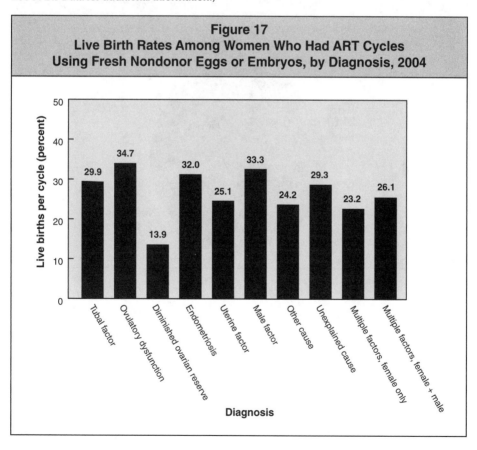

Figure 17
Live Birth Rates Among Women Who Had ART Cycles Using Fresh Nondonor Eggs or Embryos, by Diagnosis, 2004

How many women who use ART have previously given birth?

Figure 18 shows the number of previous births among women who had an ART procedure using fresh nondonor eggs or embryos in 2004. Most of these women (about 72%) had no previous births, although they may have had a pregnancy that resulted in a miscarriage or an induced abortion. About 21% of women using ART in 2004 reported one previous birth, and 7% reported two or more previous births. However, we do not have information about how many of these were ART births and how many were not. These data nonetheless point out that women who have previously had children can still face infertility problems.

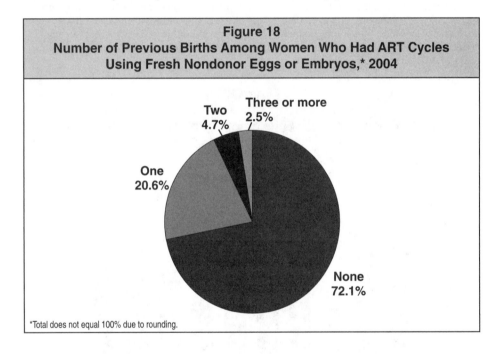

Figure 18
Number of Previous Births Among Women Who Had ART Cycles Using Fresh Nondonor Eggs or Embryos,* 2004

Two 4.7% Three or more 2.5% One 20.6% None 72.1%

*Total does not equal 100% due to rounding.

Do women who have previously given birth have higher ART success rates?

Figure 19 shows the relationship between the success of an ART cycle and the history of previous births. Previous live-born infants were conceived naturally in some cases and through ART in others. In all age groups, women who had a previous live birth were more likely to have a successful ART procedure.

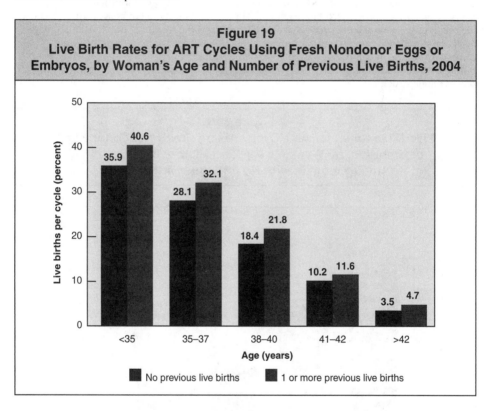

Figure 19
Live Birth Rates for ART Cycles Using Fresh Nondonor Eggs or Embryos, by Woman's Age and Number of Previous Live Births, 2004

Is there a difference in ART success rates between women with previous miscarriages and women who have never been pregnant?

In 2004, 67,983 ART cycles were performed among women who had not previously given birth. However, about 27% of those cycles were reported by women with one or more previous pregnancies that had ended in miscarriage. We do not have information on whether the previous pregnancies were the result of ART or were conceived naturally. Figure 20 shows the relationship between the success of an ART cycle and the history of previous miscarriage. In all age groups women who had a previous miscarriage had live birth rates that were comparable to the live birth rates among women who had never been pregnant. Thus, a history of unsuccessful pregnancy does not appear to be associated with reduced chances for success during ART.

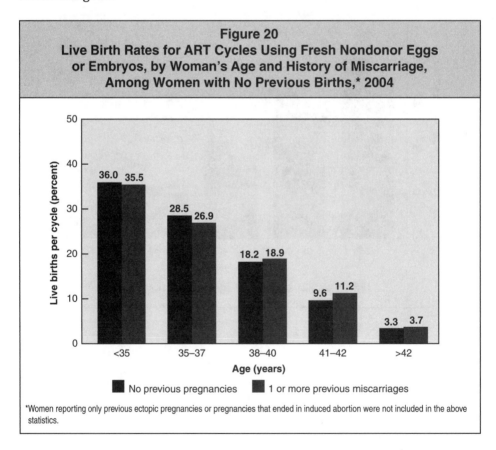

Figure 20
Live Birth Rates for ART Cycles Using Fresh Nondonor Eggs or Embryos, by Woman's Age and History of Miscarriage, Among Women with No Previous Births,* 2004

*Women reporting only previous ectopic pregnancies or pregnancies that ended in induced abortion were not included in the above statistics.

How many current ART users have undergone previous ART cycles?

Figure 21 presents ART cycles that used fresh nondonor eggs or embryos in 2004 according to whether previous ART cycles had been performed. For about 44%, one or more previous cycles were reported. (This percentage includes previous cycles using either fresh or frozen embryos.) This finding illustrates that it is not uncommon for a couple to undergo multiple ART cycles. We do not have information on when previous cycles were performed, nor do we have information on the outcomes of those previous cycles.

Figure 21
Number of Previous ART Cycles Among Women Undergoing ART in 2004 with Fresh Nondonor Eggs or Embryos

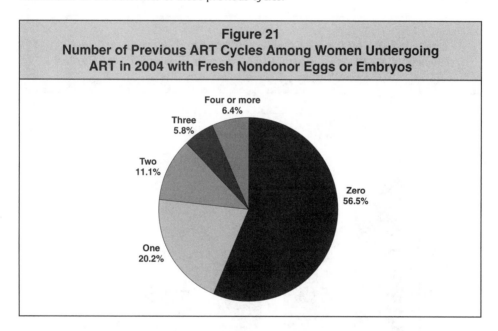

Are success rates different for women using ART for the first time and women who previously used ART but did not give birth?

Figure 22 shows the relationship between the success of ART cycles performed in 2004 using fresh nondonor eggs or embryos and a history of previous ART cycles among women with no previous births. In all age groups, success rates were lower for women who had previously undergone an unsuccessful ART cycle.

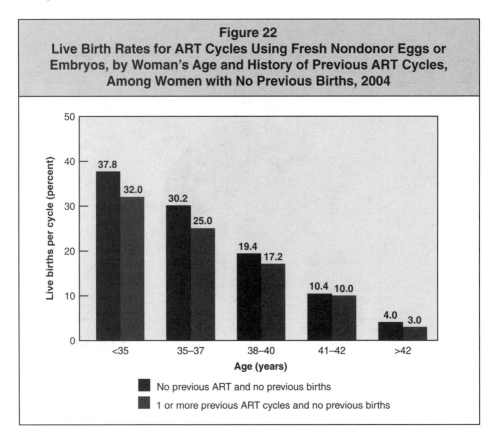

Figure 22
Live Birth Rates for ART Cycles Using Fresh Nondonor Eggs or Embryos, by Woman's Age and History of Previous ART Cycles, Among Women with No Previous Births, 2004

What are the success rates for women who have had *both* previous ART and previous births?

Figure 23 shows the relationship between the success of ART cycles performed in 2004 using fresh nondonor eggs or embryos and a history of both previous ART cycles and previous births. We do not have information on whether the previous births were the result of ART or were conceived naturally. However, among women with previous births, success rates were comparable if they had undergone previous ART cycles.

Taken together, Figures 22 and 23 show that having undergone previous ART cycles may be related to the success of the current ART cycle. However, it is important to consider the outcomes of previous cycles and whether the woman has given birth in the past.

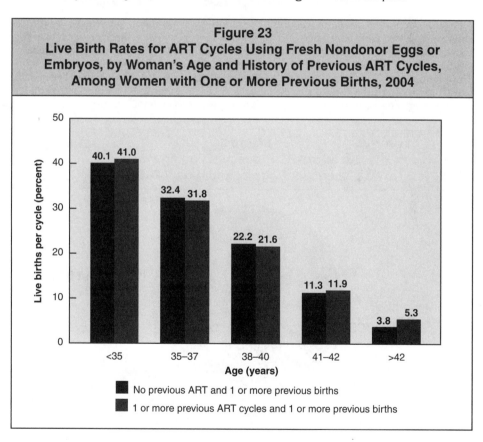

Figure 23
Live Birth Rates for ART Cycles Using Fresh Nondonor Eggs or Embryos, by Woman's Age and History of Previous ART Cycles, Among Women with One or More Previous Births, 2004

■ No previous ART and 1 or more previous births
■ 1 or more previous ART cycles and 1 or more previous births

What were the specific types of ART performed among women who used fresh nondonor eggs or embryos in 2004?

For about 42% of ART procedures that used fresh nondonor eggs or embryos in 2004, standard IVF (in vitro fertilization) techniques were used: eggs and sperm were combined in the laboratory, the resulting embryos were cultured for 2 or more days, and one or more embryos were then transferred into the woman's uterus through the cervix.

For more than half (58%) of ART procedures, fertilization was accomplished using intracytoplasmic sperm injection (ICSI). This technique involves injecting a single sperm directly into an egg; the embryos are then cultured and transferred as in standard IVF.

For a small proportion of ART procedures, unfertilized eggs and sperm (gametes) or early embryos (zygotes) were transferred into the woman's fallopian tubes. These procedures are known as gamete and zygote intrafallopian transfer (GIFT and ZIFT). Some women with tubal infertility are not suitable candidates for GIFT and ZIFT. GIFT and ZIFT are more invasive procedures than IVF because they involve inserting a laparoscope into a woman's abdomen to transfer the embryos or gametes into the fallopian tubes. In contrast, IVF involves transferring embryos or gametes into a woman's uterus through the cervix without surgery.

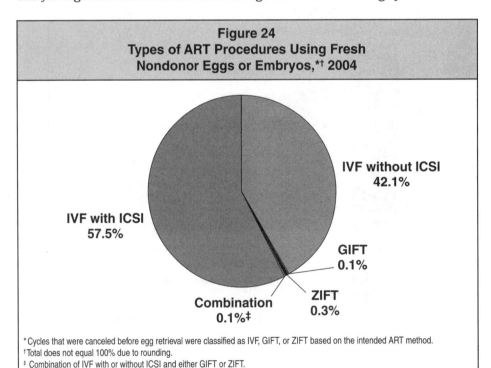

**Figure 24
Types of ART Procedures Using Fresh
Nondonor Eggs or Embryos,*† 2004**

IVF without ICSI
42.1%

IVF with ICSI
57.5%

GIFT
0.1%

ZIFT
0.3%

Combination
0.1%‡

* Cycles that were canceled before egg retrieval were classified as IVF, GIFT, or ZIFT based on the intended ART method.
† Total does not equal 100% due to rounding.
‡ Combination of IVF with or without ICSI and either GIFT or ZIFT.

What are the success rates for different types of ART procedures?

Figure 25 shows the percentage of egg retrievals that resulted in a live birth for each type of ART procedure started in 2004. Success rates for the two predominant types of ART, IVF without ICSI and IVF with ICSI, were similar. The success rates for cycles that used GIFT were much lower than for cycles that used other ART procedures. See Figures 26–28 for further details on IVF procedures that used ICSI.

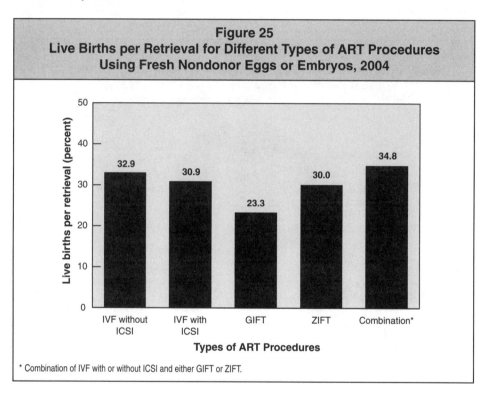

Figure 25
Live Births per Retrieval for Different Types of ART Procedures Using Fresh Nondonor Eggs or Embryos, 2004

* Combination of IVF with or without ICSI and either GIFT or ZIFT.

Is ICSI used only for couples diagnosed with male factor infertility?

ICSI was developed to overcome problems with fertilization that sometimes occur in couples diagnosed with male factor infertility. In 2004, 54,203 ICSI cycles were performed. Although the majority of couples using ICSI had a diagnosis of male factor infertility, a sizable portion of ICSI cycles (about 49%) were performed for couples without a diagnosis of male factor infertility. However, please note that diagnostic procedures may vary from one clinic to another, so the categorization of causes of infertility may also vary.

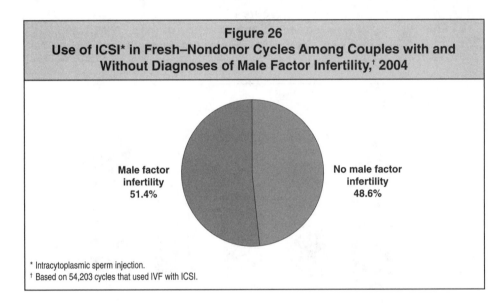

Figure 26
Use of ICSI* in Fresh–Nondonor Cycles Among Couples with and Without Diagnoses of Male Factor Infertility,[†] 2004

Male factor
infertility
51.4%

No male factor
infertility
48.6%

* Intracytoplasmic sperm injection.
[†] Based on 54,203 cycles that used IVF with ICSI.

What are the success rates for couples with male factor infertility when ICSI is used?

ICSI was developed to overcome problems with fertilization that sometimes occur in couples diagnosed with male factor infertility. In 2004, about 80% of couples diagnosed with male factor infertility used IVF with ICSI. Figure 27 presents the success rates for these ICSI procedures among couples diagnosed with male factor infertility. For comparison, these rates are presented alongside the success rates for ART cycles that used standard IVF without ICSI. This standard IVF comparison group includes couples with all diagnoses except male factor. Because ICSI can be performed only when at least one egg has been retrieved, the live birth per retrieval rates are presented.

In every age group, success rates for the IVF with ICSI group were similar to the success rates for the groups that used standard IVF without ICSI. These results show that when ICSI was used for couples diagnosed with male factor infertility, their success rates were close to those achieved by couples who were not diagnosed with male factor infertility. Please note, however, that review of select clinical records revealed that reporting of infertility causes may be incomplete. Therefore, differences in success rates by causes of infertility should be interpreted with caution. (See Findings from Validation Visits for 2004 ART Data for additional information.)

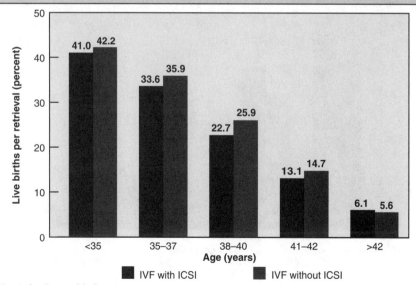

Figure 27
Live Births per Retrieval for ART Cycles Using Fresh Nondonor Eggs or Embryos Among Couples Diagnosed with Male Factor Infertility Who Used IVF with ICSI,* Compared with Couples Not Diagnosed with Male Factor Infertility Who Used IVF Without ICSI, by Woman's Age,† 2004

* Intracytoplasmic sperm injection.
† Cycles using donor sperm and cycles using GIFT and ZIFT are excluded. The comparison group of IVF without ICSI includes couples with all diagnoses except male factor infertility.

What are the success rates for couples without a diagnosis of male factor infertility when ICSI is used?

As shown in Figure 26, a large number of ICSI procedures are now performed even when couples are not diagnosed with male factor infertility. Figure 28 presents success rates per retrieval for those cycles compared with ART cycles among couples who used IVF without ICSI. For every age group, the ICSI procedures were less successful. Please note, however, that review of select clinical records revealed that reporting of infertility causes may be incomplete. Therefore, differences in success rates by causes of infertility should be interpreted with caution. (See Findings from Validation Visits for 2004 ART Data for additional information.) Additionally, information was not available to completely determine whether this finding was directly related to the ICSI procedure or whether the patients who used ICSI were somehow different from those who use IVF alone. However, separate evaluation of various groups of patients with an indication of being difficult to treat revealed a pattern of results consistent with those presented below. These difficult-to-treat groups included couples with previous failed ART cycles, couples diagnosed with diminished ovarian reserve, and couples with a low number of eggs retrieved (fewer than five). Within each of these groups, ART cycles that used IVF with ICSI had lower success rates compared with cycles that used IVF without ICSI.

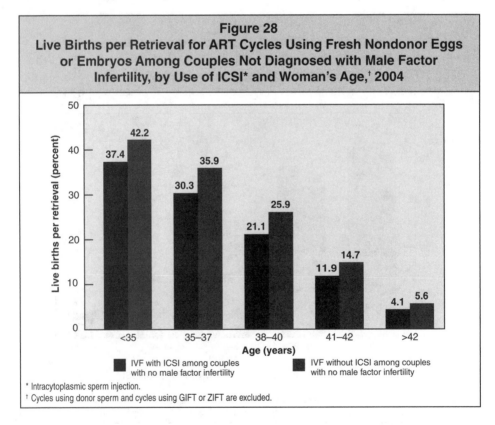

Figure 28
Live Births per Retrieval for ART Cycles Using Fresh Nondonor Eggs or Embryos Among Couples Not Diagnosed with Male Factor Infertility, by Use of ICSI* and Woman's Age,[†] 2004

Legend:
- IVF with ICSI among couples with no male factor infertility
- IVF without ICSI among couples with no male factor infertility

* Intracytoplasmic sperm injection.
[†] Cycles using donor sperm and cycles using GIFT or ZIFT are excluded.

How many embryos are transferred in an ART procedure?

Figure 29 shows that approximately 52% of ART cycles that used fresh nondonor eggs or embryos and progressed to the embryo transfer stage in 2004 involved the transfer of three or more embryos, about 21% of cycles involved the transfer of four or more, and approximately 7% of cycles involved the transfer of five or more embryos.

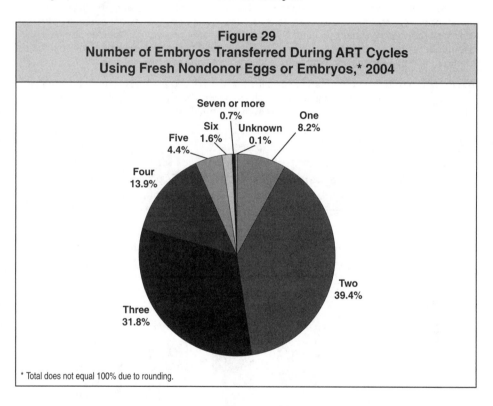

**Figure 29
Number of Embryos Transferred During ART Cycles
Using Fresh Nondonor Eggs or Embryos,* 2004**

* Total does not equal 100% due to rounding.

In general, is an ART cycle more likely to be successful if more embryos are transferred?

Figure 30 shows the relationship between the number of embryos transferred during an ART procedure in 2004 and the number of infants born alive as a result of that procedure. The success rate increased when two or more embryos were transferred; however, transferring multiple embryos also poses a risk of having a multiple-infant birth. Multiple-infant births cause concern because of the additional health risks they create for both mothers and infants. Also, pregnancies with multiple fetuses can be associated with the possibility of multifetal reduction. Multifetal reduction can happen naturally (e.g., fetal death), or a woman may decide to reduce the number of fetuses using a procedure called multifetal pregnancy reduction. Information on medical multifetal pregnancy reductions is incomplete and therefore not provided here.

The relationships between number of embryos transferred, success rates, and multiple-infant births are complicated by several factors, such as the woman's age and embryo quality. See Figure 31 for more details on women most at risk for multiple births.

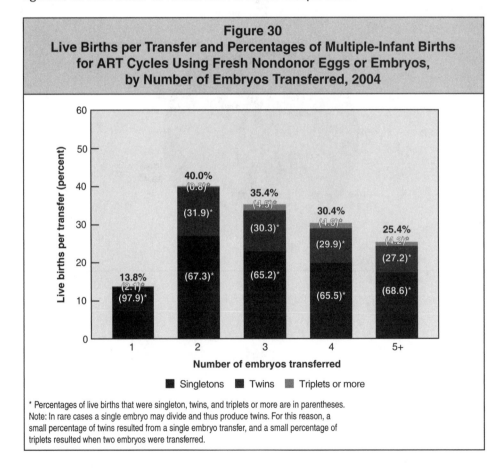

Figure 30
Live Births per Transfer and Percentages of Multiple-Infant Births for ART Cycles Using Fresh Nondonor Eggs or Embryos, by Number of Embryos Transferred, 2004

* Percentages of live births that were singleton, twins, and triplets or more are in parentheses.
Note: In rare cases a single embryo may divide and thus produce twins. For this reason, a small percentage of twins resulted from a single embryo transfer, and a small percentage of triplets resulted when two embryos were transferred.

Are live birth rates affected by the number of embryos transferred for women who have more embryos available than they choose to transfer?

Although, in general, transferring more than one embryo tends to improve the chance for a successful ART procedure (see Figure 30), other factors are also important. Previous research suggests that the number of embryos fertilized and thus available for ART is just as, if not more, important in predicting success as the number of embryos transferred. Additionally, younger women tend to have both higher success rates and higher multiple-infant birth rates. Figure 31 shows the relationship between the number of embryos transferred, success rates, and multiple-infant births for a subset of ART procedures in which the woman was younger than 35 and the couple chose to set aside some embryos for future cycles rather than transfer all available embryos at one time.

For this group, the chance for a live birth using ART was about 45% when only one embryo was transferred. If one measures success as the singleton live birth rate, the highest rate was observed with one embryo transferred.

The proportion of live births that were multiple-infant births was about 38% with two embryos and about 46% with three embryos. Transferring three or more embryos also created an additional risk for higher-order multiple births (i.e., triplets or more).

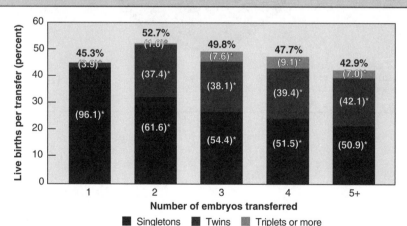

Figure 31
Live Births per Transfer and Percentages of Multiple-Infant Births for ART Cycles in Women Who Were Younger Than 35, Used Fresh Nondonor Eggs or Embryos, and Set Aside Extra Embryos for Future Use, by Number of Embryos Transferred, 2004

* Percentages of live births that were singleton, twins, and triplets or more are in parentheses.
Note: In rare cases a single embryo may divide and thus produce twins. For this reason, a small percentage of twins resulted from a single embryo transfer, and a small percentage of triplets resulted when two embryos were transferred.

How long after egg retrieval does embryo transfer occur?

Once an ART cycle has progressed from egg retrieval to fertilization, the embryo(s) can be transferred into the woman's uterus in the subsequent 1 to 6 days. Figure 32 shows that in 2004 approximately 72% of embryo transfers occurred on day 3. Day 5 embryo transfers were the next most common, accounting for about 19% of ART procedures that progressed to the embryo transfer stage.

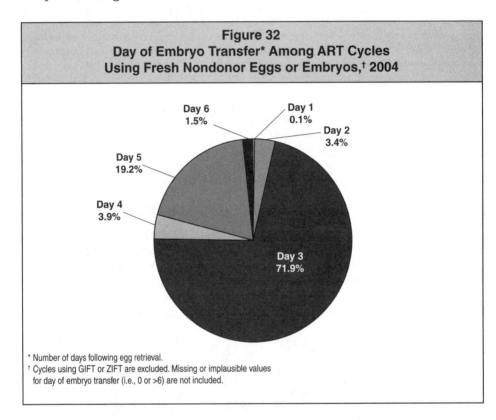

Figure 32
Day of Embryo Transfer* Among ART Cycles
Using Fresh Nondonor Eggs or Embryos,† 2004

Day 6
1.5%

Day 1
0.1%

Day 2
3.4%

Day 5
19.2%

Day 4
3.9%

Day 3
71.9%

* Number of days following egg retrieval.
† Cycles using GIFT or ZIFT are excluded. Missing or implausible values for day of embryo transfer (i.e., 0 or >6) are not included.

In general, is an ART cycle more likely to be successful if embryos are transferred on day 5?

As shown in Figure 32, in the vast majority of ART procedures, embryos were transferred on day 3 (72%) or day 5 (19%). Figure 33 compares success rates for day 3 embryo transfers with those for day 5 embryo transfers. In all age groups, the success rates were higher for day 5 embryo transfers than for day 3 transfers. However, it should be noted that day 5 embryo transfers may not be the best treatment option for all patients undergoing ART because some embryos may not survive to day 5.

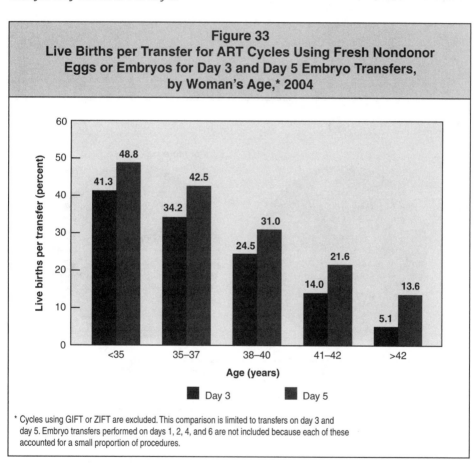

Figure 33
Live Births per Transfer for ART Cycles Using Fresh Nondonor Eggs or Embryos for Day 3 and Day 5 Embryo Transfers, by Woman's Age,* 2004

* Cycles using GIFT or ZIFT are excluded. This comparison is limited to transfers on day 3 and day 5. Embryo transfers performed on days 1, 2, 4, and 6 are not included because each of these accounted for a small proportion of procedures.

Does the number of embryos transferred differ for day 3 and day 5 embryo transfers?

Figure 34 shows the number of embryos transferred on day 3 and day 5. Overall, fewer embryos were transferred on day 5 than on day 3. Approximately 60% of day 3 embryo transfers and 25% of day 5 embryo transfers involved the transfer of three or more embryos. The decrease in the number of embryos transferred on day 5, however, did not translate into a lower risk for multiple-infant births. See Figure 35 for more details on the relationship between multiple-infant birth risk and day of embryo transfer.

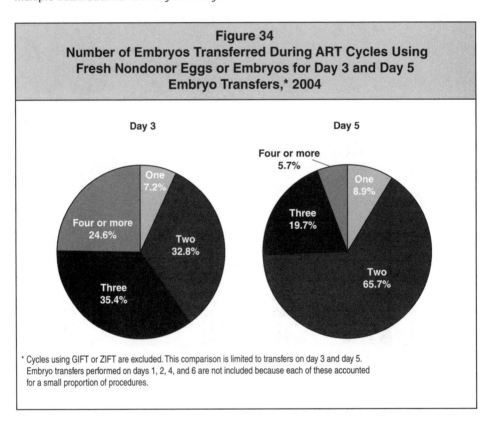

Figure 34
Number of Embryos Transferred During ART Cycles Using Fresh Nondonor Eggs or Embryos for Day 3 and Day 5 Embryo Transfers,* 2004

Day 3

Day 5

* Cycles using GIFT or ZIFT are excluded. This comparison is limited to transfers on day 3 and day 5. Embryo transfers performed on days 1, 2, 4, and 6 are not included because each of these accounted for a small proportion of procedures.

In general, how does the multiple-birth risk vary by the day of embryo transfer?

Multiple-infant births are associated with greater problems for both mothers and infants, including higher rates of caesarean section, prematurity, low birth weight, and infant disability or death.

Part A of Figure 35 shows that among the 17,634 live births that occurred following day 3 embryo transfer, 69% were singletons, 29% were twins, and about 3% were triplets or more. Thus, approximately 31% of these live births produced more than one infant.

In 2004, 6,297 live births occurred following day 5 embryo transfer. Part B of Figure 35 shows that 37% of these live births produced more than one infant (approximately 35% twins and 2% triplets or more).

As shown in Figure 34, fewer embryos were transferred on day 5 than on day 3. While the reduction in the number of embryos transferred on day 5 was associated with a decrease in triplet or more births, it also was associated with an increase in twin births. Thus, the risk of having a multiple-infant birth was higher for day 5 embryo transfers. Multiple-infant birth rates for both day 3 and day 5 embryo transfers are much higher overall than those found in the general U.S. population (about 3%).

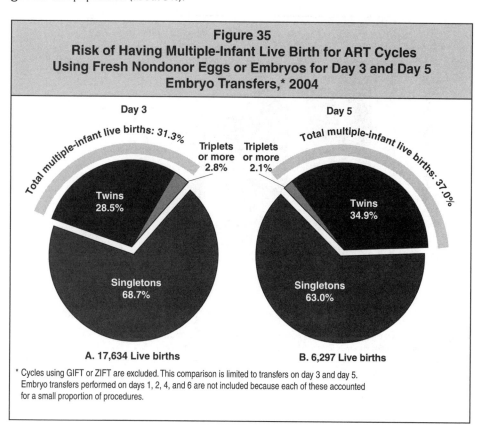

Figure 35
Risk of Having Multiple-Infant Live Birth for ART Cycles Using Fresh Nondonor Eggs or Embryos for Day 3 and Day 5 Embryo Transfers,* 2004

Day 3

Total multiple-infant live births: 31.3%

Triplets or more 2.8%   Triplets or more 2.1%

Twins 28.5%

Singletons 68.7%

A. 17,634 Live births

Day 5

Total multiple-infant live births: 37.0%

Twins 34.9%

Singletons 63.0%

B. 6,297 Live births

* Cycles using GIFT or ZIFT are excluded. This comparison is limited to transfers on day 3 and day 5. Embryo transfers performed on days 1, 2, 4, and 6 are not included because each of these accounted for a small proportion of procedures.

What are the success rates for women who use gestational carriers?

In some cases a woman has trouble carrying a pregnancy. In such cases the couple may use ART with a gestational carrier, sometimes called a surrogate. A gestational carrier is a woman who agrees to carry the developing embryo for a couple with infertility problems (the intended parents). Gestational carriers were used in 0.8% of ART cycles using fresh nondonor embryos in 2004 (710 cycles). Figure 36 compares success rates per transfer for ART cycles that used a gestational carrier in 2004 with cycles that did not. In all age groups, success rates for ART cycles that used gestational carriers were higher than success rates for those cycles that did not.

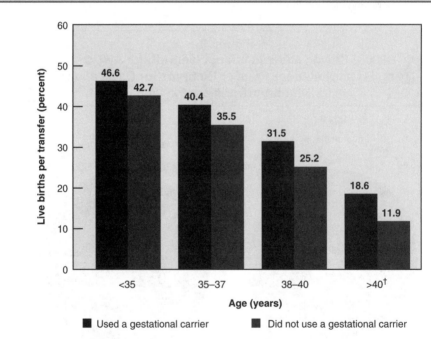

Figure 36
Comparison of Live Births per Transfer Between Cycles That Used Gestational Carriers and Those That Did Not (Both Using Fresh Nondonor Embryos), by ART Patient's Age,* 2004

* Age categories reflect the age of the ART patient, not the age of the gestational carrier.
† We were unable to further subdivide ages >40 because the number of such cycles is very small.

How is clinic size related to success rates?

The number of ART procedures carried out every year varies among fertility clinics in the United States. In 2004, success rates were similar for all clinics regardless of the number of cycles performed. For Figure 37, clinics were divided equally into four groups (called quartiles) based on the size of the clinic as determined by the number of cycles it carried out. The percentage for each quartile represents the average success rate for clinics in that quartile. For the exact number of cycles and success rates at an individual clinic, refer to the clinic table section of this report.

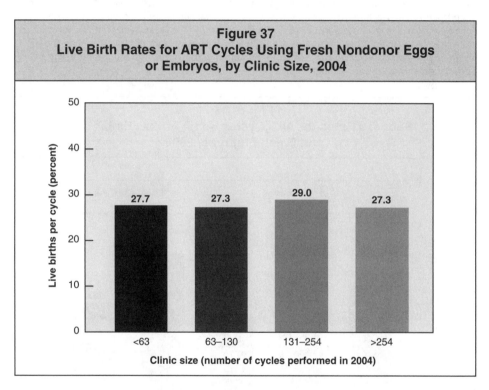

Figure 37
Live Birth Rates for ART Cycles Using Fresh Nondonor Eggs or Embryos, by Clinic Size, 2004

SECTION 3: ART CYCLES USING FROZEN NONDONOR EMBRYOS

What are the success rates for ART cycles using frozen nondonor embryos?

Frozen embryos were used in approximately 14% of all ART cycles performed in 2004 (18,560 cycles). Figure 38 compares the success rates for frozen embryos with the success rates for fresh embryos among women using their own eggs. Because some embryos do not survive the thawing process, the live birth per thaw rate is usually lower than the live birth per transfer rate. In 2004, the success rates for frozen embryos were lower than the success rates for fresh embryos. However, the average number of embryos transferred was similar for cycles using both frozen embryos and fresh embryos (see the national summary table on page 81 for information on the average number of embryos transferred for these cycles). It is important to note that cycles using frozen embryos are both less expensive and less invasive than those using fresh embryos because the woman does not have to go through the fertility drug stimulation and egg retrieval steps again.

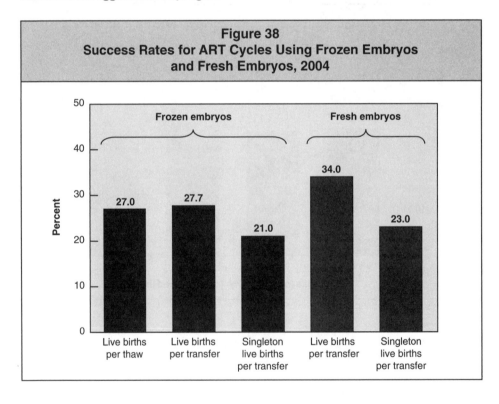

Figure 38
Success Rates for ART Cycles Using Frozen Embryos and Fresh Embryos, 2004

What is the risk of having a multiple-fetus pregnancy or multiple-infant live birth from an ART cycle using frozen nondonor embryos?

Multiple-infant births are associated with greater problems for both mothers and infants, including higher rates of caesarean section, prematurity, low birth weight, and infant disability or death.

Part A of Figure 39 shows that among the 5,898 pregnancies that resulted from ART cycles using frozen nondonor embryos, about 67% were singleton pregnancies, about 20% were twins, and nearly 4% were triplets or more. Nine percent of pregnancies ended in miscarriage before the number of fetuses could be accurately determined. Therefore, the percentage of pregnancies with more than one fetus might have been higher than what was reported (about 24%).

In 2004, 4,658 pregnancies from ART cycles that used frozen nondonor embryos resulted in live births. Part B of Figure 39 shows that approximately 24% of these live births produced more than one infant (about 22% twins and 2% triplets or more). This compares with a multiple-infant birth rate of slightly more than 3% in the general U.S. population.

Although the total rates for multiples were similar for pregnancies and live births, there were more triplet (or more) pregnancies than births. Triplet (or more) pregnancies may be reduced to twins or singletons by the time of birth. This can happen naturally (e.g., fetal death), or a woman and her doctor may decide to reduce the number of fetuses using a procedure called multifetal pregnancy reduction. Information on medical multifetal pregnancy reductions is incomplete and therefore is not provided here.

Figure 39
Risk of Having Multiple-Fetus Pregnancy and Multiple-Infant Live Birth from ART Cycles Using Frozen Nondonor Embryos, 2004

Total multiple-fetus pregnancies: 24.1%

Triplets or more 3.8%

Twins 20.3%

Not able to determine number of fetuses* 9.1%

Singletons 66.8%

A. 5,898 Pregnancies

Total multiple-infant live births: 24.2%

Triplets or more 2.1%

Twins 22.1%

Singletons 75.8%

B. 4,658 Live births

* Number of fetuses not known because the pregnancy ended in an early miscarriage.

SECTION 4: ART CYCLES USING DONOR EGGS

Are older women undergoing ART more likely to use donor eggs or embryos?

As shown in Figures 12, 13, and 14, eggs produced by women in older age groups form embryos that are less likely to implant and more likely to spontaneously abort if they do implant. As a result, ART using donor eggs is much more common among older women than among younger women. Donor eggs or embryos were used in approximately 12% of all ART cycles carried out in 2004 (15,175 cycles). Figure 40 shows the percentage of ART cycles using donor eggs in 2004 according to the woman's age. Few women younger than age 39 used donor eggs; however, the percentage of cycles carried out with donor eggs increased sharply starting at age 39. Among women older than age 47, about 91% of all ART cycles used donor eggs.

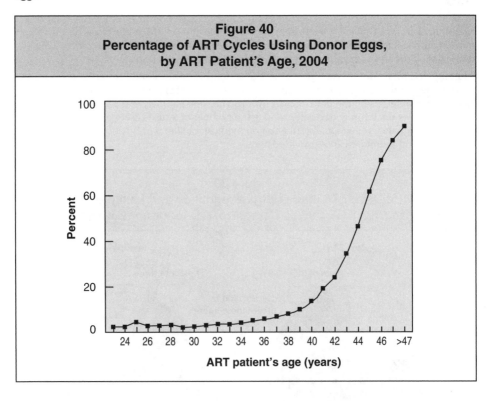

Figure 40
Percentage of ART Cycles Using Donor Eggs, by ART Patient's Age, 2004

Do success rates differ by age for women who used ART with donor eggs compared with women who used ART with their own eggs?

Figure 41 compares live birth rates for ART cycles using fresh embryos from donor eggs with those for ART cycles using a woman's own eggs among women of different ages. The likelihood of a fertilized egg implanting is related to the age of the woman who produced the egg. Egg donors are typically in their 20s or early 30s. Thus, the live birth per transfer rate for cycles using embryos from donor eggs varies only slightly across all age groups. The average live birth per transfer rate is 51%. In contrast, the live birth rates for cycles using embryos from women's own eggs decline steadily as women get older.

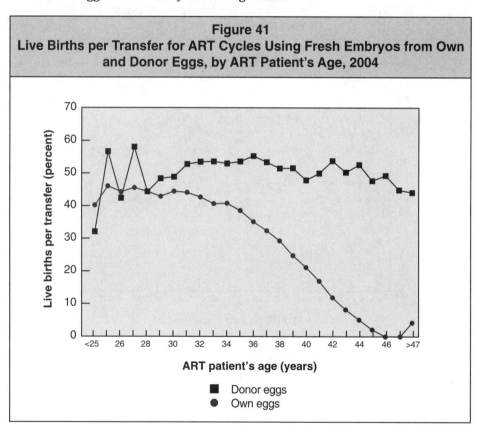

Figure 41
Live Births per Transfer for ART Cycles Using Fresh Embryos from Own and Donor Eggs, by ART Patient's Age, 2004

How successful is ART when donor eggs are used?

Figure 42 shows live birth per transfer rates and singleton live birth per transfer rates for ART cycles using fresh embryos from donor eggs among women of different ages. For all ages, the singleton live birth rates (average 30%) were lower than the total live birth rates (average 51%). Singleton live births are an important measure of success because they have a much lower risk than multiple-infant births for adverse infant health outcomes, including prematurity, low birth weight, disability, and death.

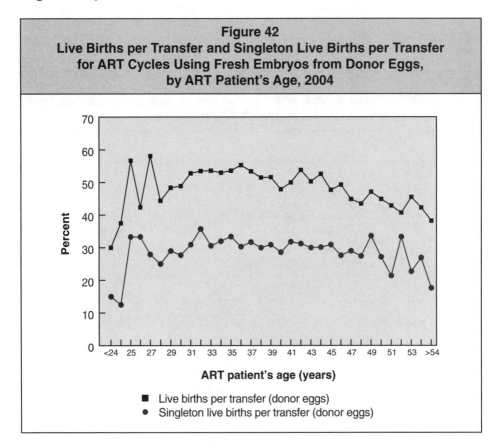

Figure 42
Live Births per Transfer and Singleton Live Births per Transfer for ART Cycles Using Fresh Embryos from Donor Eggs, by ART Patient's Age, 2004

What is the risk of having a multiple-fetus pregnancy or multiple-infant live birth from an ART cycle using fresh donor eggs?

Multiple-infant births are associated with greater problems for both mothers and infants, including higher rates of caesarean section, prematurity, low birth weight, and infant disability or death.

Part A of Figure 43 shows that among the 5,449 pregnancies that resulted from ART cycles using fresh embryos from donor eggs, about 53% were singleton pregnancies, about 37% were twins, and nearly 5% were triplets or more. About 5% of pregnancies ended in miscarriage before the number of fetuses could be accurately determined. Therefore, the percentage of pregnancies with more than one fetus might have been higher than what was reported (about 42%).

In 2004, 4,690 pregnancies from ART cycles that used fresh embryos from donor eggs resulted in live births. Part B of Figure 43 shows that 40% of these live births produced more than one infant (about 38% twins and about 2% triplets or more). This compares with a multiple-infant birth rate of slightly more than 3% in the general population.

Although the total rates for multiples were similar for pregnancies and live births, there were more triplet (or more) pregnancies than births. Triplet (or more) pregnancies may be reduced to twins or singletons by the time of birth. This can happen naturally (e.g., fetal death), or a woman and her doctor may decide to reduce the number of fetuses using a procedure called multifetal pregnancy reduction. Information on medical multifetal pregnancy reductions is incomplete and therefore is not provided here.

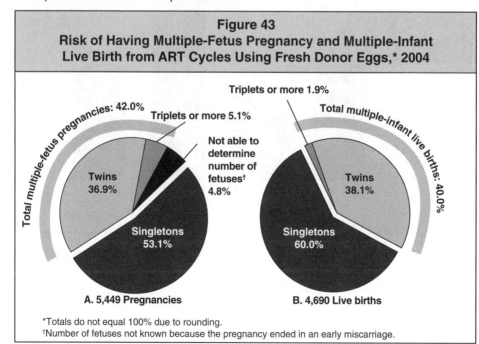

Figure 43
Risk of Having Multiple-Fetus Pregnancy and Multiple-Infant Live Birth from ART Cycles Using Fresh Donor Eggs,* 2004

Total multiple-fetus pregnancies: 42.0%
Triplets or more 5.1%
Twins 36.9%
Not able to determine number of fetuses† 4.8%
Singletons 53.1%
A. 5,449 Pregnancies

Triplets or more 1.9%
Total multiple-infant live births: 40.0%
Twins 38.1%
Singletons 60.0%
B. 4,690 Live births

*Totals do not equal 100% due to rounding.
†Number of fetuses not known because the pregnancy ended in an early miscarriage.

How do success rates differ between women who use frozen donor embryos and those who use fresh donor embryos?

Figure 44 shows that the success rates per transfer for frozen donor embryos were substantially lower than the success rates per transfer for fresh donor embryos. This is similar to the findings for frozen nondonor embryos (see Figure 38, page 50). The average number of embryos transferred was similar for cycles using frozen donor embryos and those using fresh donor embryos. (See the national summary table on page 81 for information on the average number of embryos transferred for these cycles.)

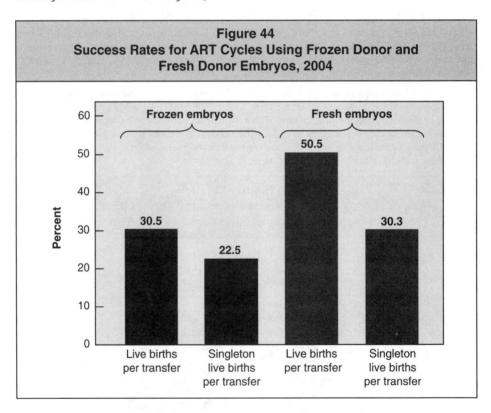

Figure 44
Success Rates for ART Cycles Using Frozen Donor and Fresh Donor Embryos, 2004

SECTION 5: ART TRENDS, 1996–2004

This report marks the tenth consecutive year that CDC has published an annual report detailing the success rates for ART clinics in the United States. Having several years of data provides us with the opportunity to examine trends in ART use and success rates over time. Because the first year of data collection, 1995, did not include non-SART member clinics, we limit our examination of trends to the years 1996–2004.

Is the use of ART increasing?

Figure 45 shows the numbers of ART cycles performed, live-birth deliveries, and infants born using ART from 1996 through 2004. The number of ART cycles performed in the United States has almost doubled, from 64,681 cycles in 1996 to 127,977 in 2004. The number of live-birth deliveries in 2004 (36,760) was about two and a half times higher than in 1996 (14,507). The number of infants born who were conceived using ART also increased steadily between 1996 and 2004. In 2004, 49,458 infants were born, which was more than double the 20,840 born in 1996. Because in some cases more than one infant is born during a live-birth delivery (e.g., twins), the total number of infants born is greater than the number of live-birth deliveries.

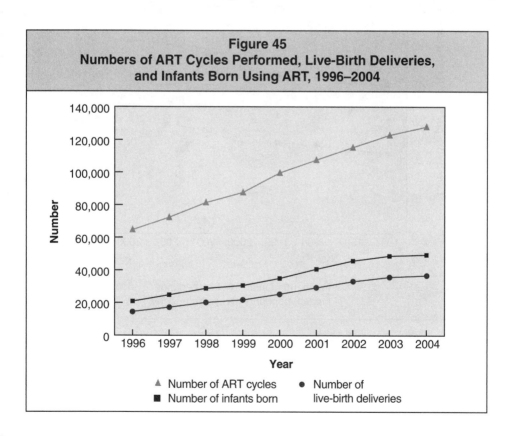

Figure 45
Numbers of ART Cycles Performed, Live-Birth Deliveries, and Infants Born Using ART, 1996–2004

Are live birth rates improving?

Figure 46 presents live birth rates for the four primary types of ART cycles. Live birth rates are presented per transfer rather than per cycle because that is the only way to directly compare cycles using fresh embryos with those using frozen embryos.

From 1996 through 2004, the live birth rates for fresh–nondonor cycles increased 21%, from 28% in 1996 to 34% in 2004. Over the same time period, live birth rates increased 47% for frozen–nondonor cycles, 30% for fresh–donor cycles, and 66% for frozen–donor cycles.

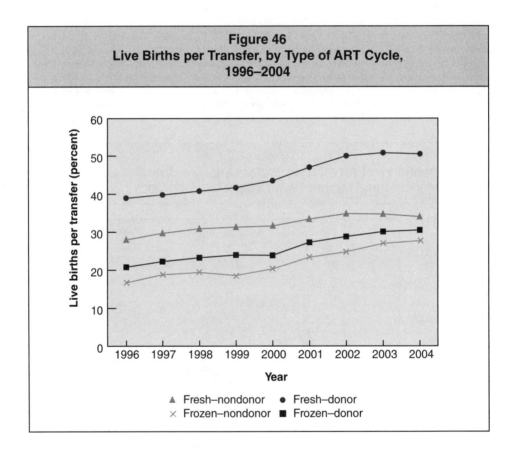

Figure 46
Live Births per Transfer, by Type of ART Cycle,
1996–2004

Are singleton live birth rates improving?

Singleton live births are an important measure of success because they have a much lower risk than multiple-infant births for adverse infant health outcomes, including prematurity, low birth weight, disability, and death. Figure 47 presents singleton live birth rates for the four primary types of ART cycles. Singleton live birth rates are presented per transfer rather than per cycle because that is the only way to directly compare cycles using fresh embryos with those using frozen embryos.

From 1996 through 2004, the singleton live birth rates for fresh–nondonor cycles increased 34%, from 17% in 1996 to 23% in 2004. Over the same time period, singleton live birth rates increased 72% for frozen–nondonor cycles, 33% for fresh–donor cycles, and 47% for frozen–donor cycles.

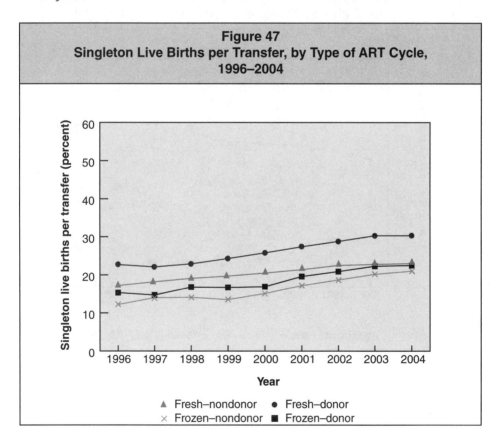

Figure 47
Singleton Live Births per Transfer, by Type of ART Cycle, 1996–2004

Are live birth rates improving for all ART patients or only for those in particular age groups?

Figure 48 presents live birth rates per transfer, by woman's age, for ART cycles using fresh nondonor eggs or embryos.

From 1996 through 2004, the live birth rates for women younger than 35 increased 27%, from 34% in 1996 to 43% in 2004. Over the same time period, live birth rates increased 22% for women 35–37, 17% for women 38–40, 29% for women 41–42, and 13% for women older than 42.

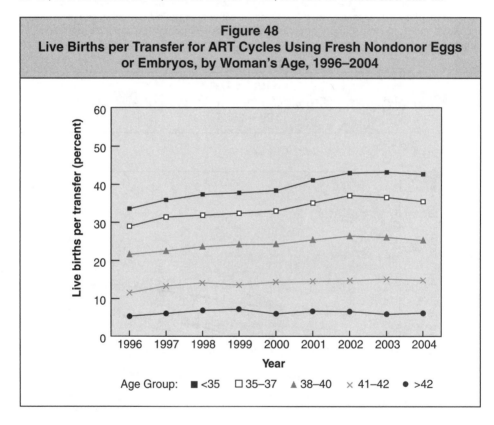

Figure 48
Live Births per Transfer for ART Cycles Using Fresh Nondonor Eggs or Embryos, by Woman's Age, 1996–2004

Age Group: ■ <35   □ 35–37   ▲ 38–40   × 41–42   ● >42

Are singleton live birth rates improving for all ART patients or only for those in particular age groups?

Singleton live births are an important measure of success because they have a much lower risk than multiple-infant births for adverse infant health outcomes, including prematurity, low birth weight, disability, and death. Figure 49 presents singleton live birth rates per transfer, by woman's age, for ART cycles using fresh nondonor eggs or embryos.

From 1996 through 2004, the singleton live birth rate for women younger than 35 increased about 41%, from 19% in 1996 to 27% in 2004. Over the same time period, live birth rates increased 33% for women 35–37, 23% for women 38–40, 29% for women 41–42, and 22% for women older than 42.

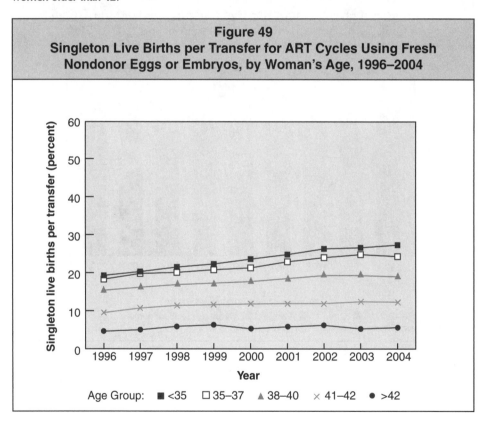

Figure 49
Singleton Live Births per Transfer for ART Cycles Using Fresh Nondonor Eggs or Embryos, by Woman's Age, 1996–2004

Has the number of embryos transferred in fresh–nondonor cycles changed?

Figure 50 presents the trends for number of embryos transferred in fresh–nondonor cycles that progressed to the embryo transfer stage. From 1996 to 2004, cycles that involved the transfer of one embryo increased slightly, from 6% to 8%; cycles that involved the transfer of two embryos increased dramatically, from 10% in 1996 to 39% in 2004. Cycles that involved the transfer of three embryos increased from 23% in 1996 to 32% in 2004, and cycles that involved the transfer of four or more embryos decreased from 62% in 1996 to 21% in 2004.

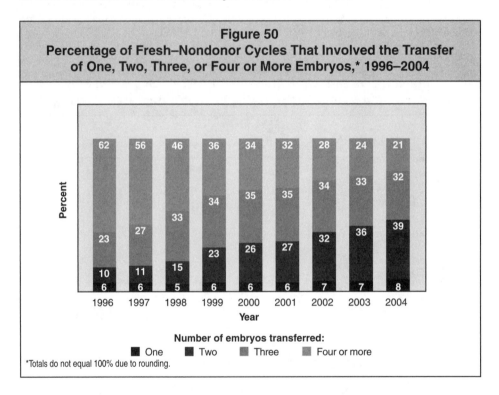

Figure 50
Percentage of Fresh–Nondonor Cycles That Involved the Transfer of One, Two, Three, or Four or More Embryos,* 1996–2004

Number of embryos transferred: ■ One ■ Two ■ Three ■ Four or more
*Totals do not equal 100% due to rounding.

Has the number of embryos transferred in each ART cycle changed for women younger than 35 who have more embryos available than they choose to transfer?

As shown in Figure 50, the number of embryos transferred in fresh–nondonor cycles has decreased during the past 9 years. Figure 51 shows the change over time in the number of embryos transferred for ART procedures in which the woman was younger than 35 and the couple chose to set aside some embryos for future cycles rather than transfer all available embryos at one time. Previous research suggests that the number of embryos available for an ART cycle is important in predicting success. Younger women also tend to have higher success rates (see Figure 31).

Overall, the number of embryos transferred decreased among couples who chose to transfer fewer embryos than were available. In 1996, almost two-thirds (64%) of ART cycles involved the transfer of four or more embryos; 33%, three embryos; and only 3%, two embryos. By 1998, the percentage of cycles in which four or more embryos were transferred had decreased to 33%; half of all ART cycles involved the transfer of three embryos, and 17% of cycles, two embryos. By 2004, four or more embryos were transferred in only 5% of cycles, three in 25% of cycles, and two in more than two-thirds (70%) of cycles.

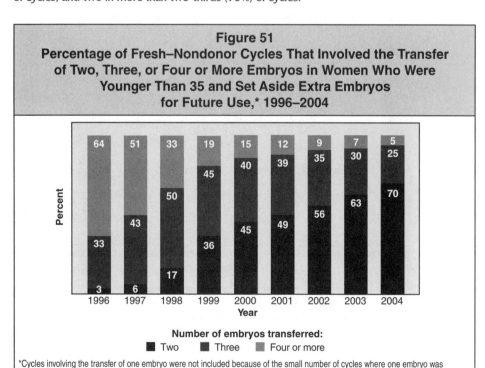

Figure 51
Percentage of Fresh–Nondonor Cycles That Involved the Transfer of Two, Three, or Four or More Embryos in Women Who Were Younger Than 35 and Set Aside Extra Embryos for Future Use,* 1996–2004

Number of embryos transferred:
■ Two ■ Three ■ Four or more

*Cycles involving the transfer of one embryo were not included because of the small number of cycles where one embryo was transferred and extra embryos were set aside for future use.

Have there been improvements in live birth rates, by number of embryos transferred?

Figure 52 presents live birth rates per transfer, by number of embryos transferred, for ART cycles using fresh nondonor eggs or embryos from 1996 through 2004. In general, the live birth rate was higher when two or more embryos were transferred. From 1996 through 2004, the live birth rate almost tripled, from 14% to 40%, for ART cycles that involved the transfer of two embryos. The live birth rates also increased for ART cycles that involved the transfer of either one or three embryos; however, live birth rates decreased 9%, from 32% to 29%, for ART cycles that involved the transfer of four or more embryos.

The relationship between number of embryos transferred and success rates is complicated by several factors, such as the woman's age and embryo quality. Trends over time may reflect changes in these factors.

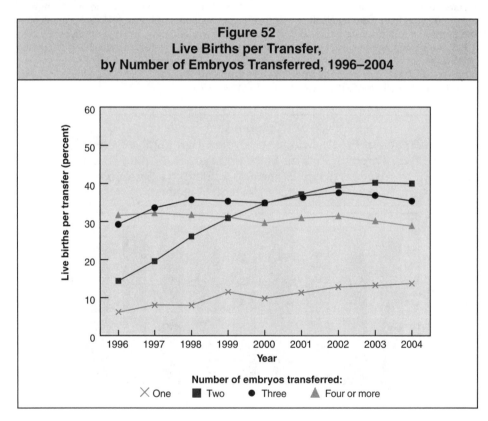

Figure 52
Live Births per Transfer,
by Number of Embryos Transferred, 1996–2004

Have live birth rates improved for women younger than 35 who have more embryos available than they choose to transfer?

Figure 53 shows changes over time in the relationship between live birth rates and number of embryos transferred for ART procedures in which the woman was younger than 35 and the couple chose to set aside some embryos for future cycles rather than transfer all available embryos at one time. Previous research suggests that the number of embryos available for an ART cycle is an important predictor of success. Younger women also tend to have higher success rates (see Figure 31).

For this group, live birth rates increased over time for transfers involving any number of embryos. The increase in success rates was largest when two embryos were transferred. In 1996, the chance for a live birth using ART was highest (41%) when three embryos were transferred; however, in 2004, the chance for a live birth using ART was highest (53%) when two embryos were transferred.

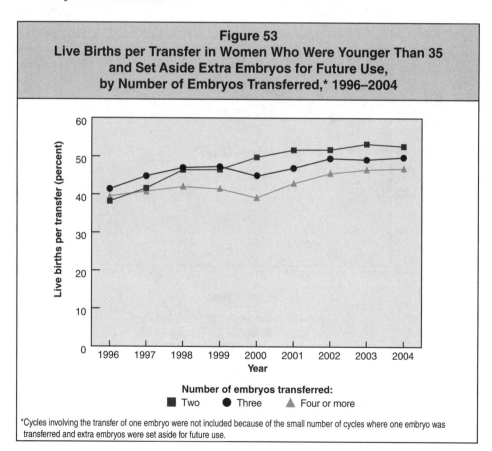

Figure 53
Live Births per Transfer in Women Who Were Younger Than 35 and Set Aside Extra Embryos for Future Use, by Number of Embryos Transferred,* 1996–2004

Number of embryos transferred:
■ Two   ● Three   ▲ Four or more

*Cycles involving the transfer of one embryo were not included because of the small number of cycles where one embryo was transferred and extra embryos were set aside for future use.

Have multiple-infant birth rates changed?

Multiple-infant births are associated with greater problems for both mothers and infants, including higher rates of caesarean section, prematurity, low birth weight, and infant disability or death. Figure 54 shows the multiple-infant birth rates for the four primary types of ART procedures.

From 1996 through 2004, the percentage of live-birth deliveries that were multiple-infant births decreased 15%, from 38% in 1996 to 33%, for fresh–nondonor cycles. Over the same time period, the percentage of live-birth deliveries that were multiple-infant births decreased 10% for frozen–nondonor cycles and 4% for fresh–donor cycles. In all years except 1997, the multiple-infant birth rates remained stable for frozen–donor cycles.

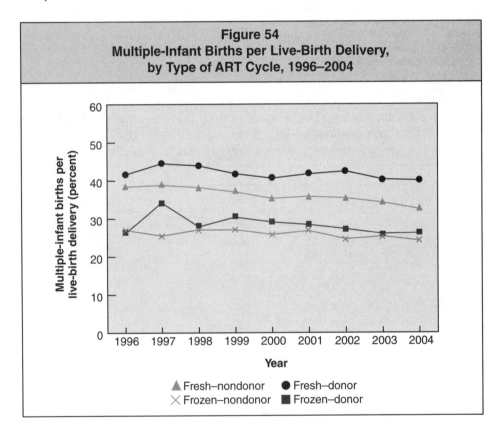

**Figure 54
Multiple-Infant Births per Live-Birth Delivery,
by Type of ART Cycle, 1996–2004**

Have multiple-infant birth rates for cycles using fresh nondonor eggs or embryos changed for all ART patients or only for those in particular age groups?

Figure 55 shows that the multiple-infant birth rates decreased slightly between 1996 and 2004 for women in all age groups. In 1996, 43% of live-birth deliveries to women younger than 35 were multiple-infant births, compared with 36% in 2004. Among women older than 42, the multiple-infant birth rates decreased from 14% in 1996 to 8% in 2004.

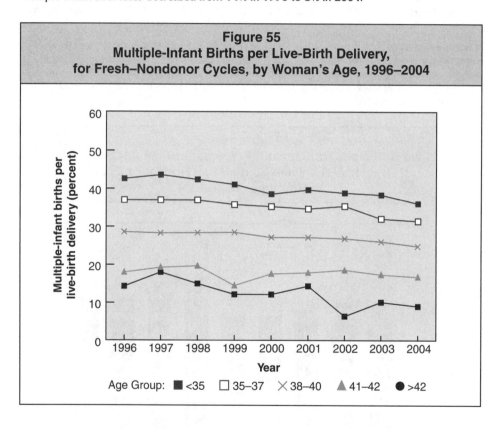

Figure 55
Multiple-Infant Births per Live-Birth Delivery,
for Fresh–Nondonor Cycles, by Woman's Age, 1996–2004

Have the percentages of singletons, twins, and triplets or more changed for ART cycles using fresh nondonor eggs or embryos?

Figure 56 presents the trends in live birth rates and percentage of multiple-infant births for ART cycles using fresh nondonor eggs or embryos. Overall, live birth rates per transfer increased from 28% in 1996 to 35% in 2003 and decreased slightly, to 34%, in 2004. From 1996 to 2004, the percentage of singleton live births increased from 62% to 67%; the percentage of twin births remained stable, ranging from 30% to 32%; and the percentage of triplet-or-more births decreased from 7% in 1996 to 3% in 2004.

It is important to note that twins, albeit to a lesser extent than triplets or more, are still at substantially greater risk for illness and death than singletons. These risks include low birth weight, preterm birth, and neurological impairments such as cerebral palsy. Both the twin and triplet-or-more birth rates remain significantly higher for ART births than for births resulting from natural conception.

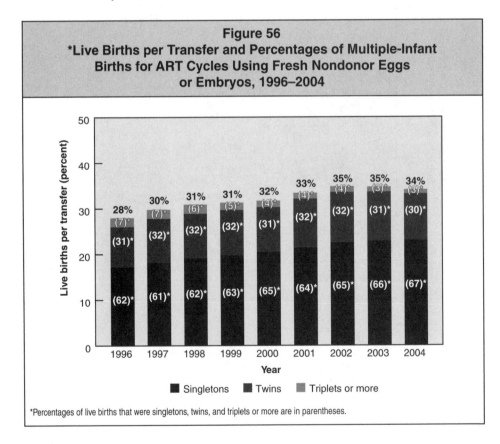

Figure 56
*Live Births per Transfer and Percentages of Multiple-Infant Births for ART Cycles Using Fresh Nondonor Eggs or Embryos, 1996–2004

*Percentages of live births that were singletons, twins, and triplets or more are in parentheses.

Glossary

A

Acanthosis nigricans: A velvety skin discoloration associated with insulin resistance.

Acrosome reaction: A test to assess the biochemical changes on the head of the sperm that may predict the ability of the sperm to fertilize an egg.

Adhesions: Bands of fibrous tissue that can bind reproductive organs, thereby reducing a woman's fertility.

Aneuploidy: Having an abnormal number of chromosomes.

Anovulation: Failure to release an egg on a regular basis, resulting in irregular or absent periods.

Anticardiolipin antibodies: Specific antibodies that are formed against various components of the cells of the body; their presence is often associated with pregnancy loss.

Antiphospholipid antibodies: The general class of antibodies that are formed against various components of the cells of the body; their presence is often associated with pregnancy loss.

Antisperm antibodies: Proteins that can lead to infertility by impairing fertilization or enhancing sperm destruction within the female reproductive tract.

Antithrombin III: A protein involved in the coagulation cascade. A deficiency in antithrombin III is associated with an increased risk of blood clotting and pregnancy loss.

Antral follicle count: The number of resting follicles seen on ultrasound early in a woman's cycle.

Artificial insemination: A group of fertility procedures involving the introduction of sperm into the female reproductive tract without intercourse.

Assisted hatching: The process of making a small hole in the shell (zona pellucida) surrounding the embryo prior to embryo transfer to promote its implantation in the uterus.

Assisted reproductive technologies (ART): A variety of fertility procedures (including in vitro fertilization) that involve manipulating sperm and eggs to achieve pregnancy.

Autosomal dominant diseases: Genetic diseases carried on a chromosome other than the X or Y chromosomes (sex chromosomes), in which a single abnormal copy of the gene leads to the presence of the disease.

Autosomal recessive diseases: Genetic diseases carried on a chromosome other than the X or Y chromosomes (sex chromosomes), in which two abnormal copies of the gene are necessary for the disease to be present.

Azoospermia: The absence of sperm in a semen analysis.

B

Balanced translocation: A chromosomal rearrangement in which two chromosomes break apart and re-form as a new chromosome containing parts of both of the original chromosomes.

Blastocyst: A stage in embryo development reached 5 days after fertilization.

Blastomeres: The individual cells present in an early cleavage-stage embryo.

Body mass index (BMI): A mathematical calculation that uses height and weight to determine whether an individual is of normal weight, overweight, or obese.

C

Chlamydia: A common sexually transmitted disease that can damage a woman's fallopian tubes.

Chromosomes: One of the threadlike "packages" of genes and other DNA in the nucleus of a cell. Humans have 23 pairs of chromosomes, for a total of 46 in all: 44 autosomes and 2 sex chromosomes.

Clomiphene citrate challenge test (CCCT): A test used to evaluate a woman's ovarian reserve before she undergoes a fertility treatment.

Congenital bilateral absence of the vas deferens (CBAVD): Absence of the sperm-carrying duct in a man, resulting in azoospermia. This condition is frequently associated with cystic fibrosis.

Controlled ovarian hyperstimulation: Stimulation of the ovaries with fertility medications to help them grow and release multiple eggs.

Corpus luteum: The hormone-producing ovarian cyst that forms from the follicle after it releases the egg.

Cryopreservation: Freezing of sperm, eggs, or embryos so as to preserve them for use at a later date.

D

Day-3 hormones: Measurement of follicle-stimulating hormone and estradiol on the second or third day of a regular menstrual cycle, which provides an assessment of a woman's ovarian reserve.

Diminished ovarian reserve: The inability to respond appropriately to fertility medications, both in terms of the number of follicles produced and the health of the eggs.

Dizygotic twins: Twins resulting from the implantation of embryos from two different eggs (also called fraternal twins).

Donor-egg IVF: An extremely successful type of in vitro fertilization procedure using the eggs from a young woman and with the resulting embryo(s) transferred into the recipient.

Dysmenorrhea: Extremely painful periods.

E

Ectopic pregnancy: A pregnancy located outside the uterine cavity, usually in the fallopian tube, though it can also occur in the ovary or abdomen (rarely).

Egg collection: A minimally invasive procedure usually performed transvaginally under minimal sedation in which eggs are removed from the ovaries.

Embryo transfer: The placement of embryos created via in vitro fertilization into the uterus or, more rarely, the fallopian tube.

Embryologist: A scientist involved in the fertilization and culture of human eggs and embryos.

Endometrial biopsy: A sample of the lining of the uterus, usually performed to rule out endometrial cancer.

Endometriomas: An ovarian cyst that is filled with chocolate-colored fluid as a result of endometriosis growing within the ovary.

Endometriosis: The presence of tissue that is usually found within the endometrial cavity in another location (most frequently on the ovaries or along the uterosacral ligaments).

Endometrium: The tissue that lines the uterine cavity and is shed each month with a woman's period.

Epididymis: Paired sac-like structures that are found atop each testicle and that serve as a repository for sperm prior to ejaculation.

Estrogen: A steroid hormone produced within the growing follicle that induces growth of the endometrium.

F

Factor V Leiden: A genetic disorder that predisposes a woman to blood clot formation and miscarriage.

Fallopian tube: The conduit that serves as an incubator following release and fertilization of the egg.

Fertilization: The process by which an egg and a sperm combine and create an embryo.

Fibroids: Benign growths of the connective tissue of the uterus that can grow quite large and cause menstrual problems, infertility, and miscarriage.

Fifth's disease: An infectious disease caused by parvovirus B19. It leads to bright rosy checks in children but can cause miscarriage if a woman contracts it during pregnancy.

Fimbria: The finger-like projections at the distal end of the fallopian tube that are responsible for trapping the egg following ovulation.

Flare stimulation protocol: A technique of follicular stimulation that begins at the start of a spontaneous menstrual cycle.

Follicles: Fluid-filled structures within the ovary that contain an egg.

Follicle-stimulating hormone (FSH): A protein hormone produced within the pituitary gland at the base of the brain that promotes the growth and development of follicles, leading eventually to ovulation.

Frozen embryo transfer (FET): Placement of previously cryopreserved embryos into the uterus or, more rarely, the fallopian tube.

Functional hypothalamic amenorrhea (FHA): The absence of menstrual cycles related to failure of the hypothalamus and pituitary gland to stimulate follicular growth.

G

Gestational carrier: A woman who undergoes an embryo transfer consisting of an embryo produced by another couple (or from donor gametes) with the intention to give the resulting baby back to the genetic parents.

Gonadotropin-releasing hormone (GnRH) analog: Medication that initially causes the pituitary gland to release its stores of follicle-stimulating hormone and luteinizing hormone, but that with continued use leads to markedly suppressed levels of these two hormones.

Gonadotropin-releasing hormone (GnRH) antagonist: Medication that quickly interferes with the production of follicle-stimulating hormone and luteinizing hormone by the pituitary gland, preventing premature ovulation during a treatment cycle.

Gonadotropins: Fertility medications containing follicle-stimulating hormone alone or in combination with luteinizing hormone that are used to induce follicle growth during fertility treatments.

Gonorrhea: A sexually transmitted disease that can cause tubal damage and infertility.

H

Heparin: An injectable medication that is used to prevent blood clot formation.

Human chorionic gonadotropin (HCG): A placental hormone produced in pregnancy that is the basis for blood and urine pregnancy testing.

Hydrosalpinx: Obstruction of the fallopian tube at the fimbria, resulting in a fluid-filled and dilated tube.

Hyperprolactinemia: Excessive secretion of the hormone prolactin.

Hypoestrogenic: A state of low estrogen.

Hypo-osmotic swelling test: A sperm test that evaluates the integrity of the outer membrane of the sperm as a means to predict the sperm's fertilizing ability.

Hysterosalpingogram: An x-ray procedure during which a radio-opaque dye is injected into the uterine cavity to assess the fallopian tubes for patency as well as the contour of the uterine cavity itself.

Hysteroscopy: A procedure allowing visualization of the uterine cavity with a small fiber-optic telescope.

Hysterosonogram: A type of transvaginal sonogram performed after placement of a small catheter into the uterine cavity through which sterile water is introduced, allowing for visualization of the uterine cavity.

I

Implantation: The attachment of the early embryo to the endometrial lining of the uterus during the seventh to ninth days after ovulation.

Incompetent cervix: A muscular-fibrous weakening of the cervix, leading to painless cervical dilation and second-trimester or early third-trimester pregnancy loss.

Infertility: The inability of a couple to conceive after 12 months of unprotected intercourse.

Insulin resistance: Impaired response to insulin, which can lead eventually to diabetes.

Intracervical insemination: A fertility treatment in which sperm are placed within the cervix.

Intracytoplasmic sperm injection (ICSI): The injection of a single sperm into a single egg in an attempt to fertilize the egg in in vitro fertilization cases when fertilization might not otherwise occur.

Intrauterine adhesions: Fibrous bands of tissue found within the uterine cavity.

Intrauterine insemination (IUI): A fertility treatment in which the sperm are washed and then placed within the uterine cavity.

In vitro fertilization (IVF): A fertility treatment in which an egg is placed with a sperm cell in a laboratory culture dish, cultured for several days, and subsequently placed into the uterus.

K

Karyotype: The chromosomal complement of an individual, including the number of chromosomes and any chromosomal abnormalities.

L

Laparoscopy: An outpatient surgical procedure that uses a telescope and video monitor to visualize the internal organs.

Laparotomy: An inpatient surgical procedure that is performed through an open abdominal incision.

Luteal suppression: A stimulation protocol that involves suppression of the pituitary gland and ovary prior to initiating stimulation with fertility medications.

Luteinizing hormone (LH): A pituitary hormone that induces ovulation in a mature follicle.

M

Macroadenoma: A tumor of the pituitary gland measuring more than 1 cm.

Menopause: The last menstrual period that a woman ever experiences.

Methyltetrahydrofolate reductase (MTHFR): An enzyme involved in folic acid metabolism.

Microadenoma: A tumor of the pituitary gland measuring less than 1 cm.

Monoamniotic twins: Monochorionic (identical) twins who share a single gestational sac. Carrying monoamniotic twins is considered to be a very high-risk pregnancy.

Monochorionic twins: Monozygotic twins who share a single placenta.

Monozygotic twins: twins arising from a single fertilized egg (also called identical twins).

Morula: An early stage of embryonic development in which the embryo consists of a solid ball of cells; the morula is formed prior to the blastocyst.

Mosaicism: The presence of both genetically normal and abnormal cells within an embryo prior to implantation.

Mycoplasma: A type of bacteria that may contribute to infertility.

O

Oligospermia: An abnormally low concentration of sperm in a semen analysis.

Oral contraceptive pills: Daily medications, usually containing both synthetic estrogen and progesterone, that act as very effective contraceptives by suppressing follicle growth and ovulation.

Osteoporosis: Loss of calcium and bone mass, leading to an increased risk of fracture.

Ovarian hyperstimulation syndrome (OHSS): Ovarian enlargement, abdominal fluid retention, and dehydration following the use of fertility medication to induce the growth of multiple follicles.

Ovarian reserve: The fertility potential of a woman as determined by both the number of her ovarian follicles and the health of the eggs located within those follicles.

Ovary: A female reproductive organ that contains eggs within multiple follicles and produces reproductive hormones including estrogen and progesterone.

Ovulation: The release of an egg from an ovarian follicle.

Ovulation induction: The use of fertility medications to restore normal ovulation in a woman who does not have regular cycles.

P

Paracentesis: Placement of a needle through the abdominal wall so as to remove excess abdominal fluid.

Parvovirus B19: A virus that can cause an intrauterine infection leading to fetal anemia, fetal heart failure, and miscarriage.

Perimenopause: The years preceding the last menstrual cycle characterized by increasingly irregular cycles, hot flashes, and low estrogen levels.

Pituitary gland: An organ located at the base of the brain. It is often referred to as the "master gland" because it controls

several of the other hormone-producing glands, including those responsible for metabolism and reproduction.

Polycystic ovarian syndrome (PCOS): A common gynecologic disorder resulting from insulin resistance and leading to irregular periods, acne, excessive facial hair, and infertility.

Postcoital test: A test of historical interest used to assess the presence and behavior of sperm found within the cervical mucus.

Preeclampsia: A vascular disease of pregnancy characterized by hypertension, edema, and a risk of seizure.

Preimplantation genetic diagnosis (PGD): Evaluation of the genetic status of an embryo prior to its implantation, usually through the removal of 1 to 2 cells at the 8-cell stage of development. The isolated cells can then be analyzed for specific chromosomal conditions and other genetic disorders.

Preimplantation genetic screening (PGS): An evaluation that is similar to preimplantation genetic diagnosis but is used to screen embryos in fertility patients for aneuploidy instead of a specific genetic disease.

Premature ovarian failure (POF): Irregular or absent menstrual cycles before the age of 40 years old, resulting from a marked loss of ovarian follicles as evidenced by a high blood level of follicle-stimulating hormone (FSH > 30 IU).

Progesterone: A steroid hormone produced by the ovary and then by the placenta during pregnancy. It is necessary for the successful implantation and development of an embryo.

Prolactin: A hormone produced by the anterior pituitary that stimulates breast milk production in a lactating woman. Inappropriate release of prolactin can cause irregular or absent menses.

Proteins C and S: Proteins involved in the blood clotting system.

Prothrombin II: A protein involved in the blood clotting system.

R

Reproductive endocrinologist: A physician who specializes in disorders of reproduction, including infertility.

Retrograde ejaculation: Backward movement of semen into the urinary bladder at the time of ejaculation.

S

Semen analysis: A laboratory test used to assess male fertility. It usually includes evaluation of the sperm volume, pH, concentration, motility and morphology in a sample.

Sperm Chromatin Structure Assay (SCSA®): A laboratory test used to determine the degree of DNA fragmentation within a sperm sample.

Sperm motility: The movement of sperm when viewed under a microscope; it is usually expressed as a percentage of the sperm concentration.

Sperm morphology: The shape and outward appearance of the sperm when viewed under a microscope.

Superovulation: The development of multiple ovarian follicles in response to fertility medication.

Systemic lupus erythematosus (lupus): A systemic autoimmune disease that causes inflammation, arthritis, rash, and other medical problems, including pregnancy loss.

T

Thrombophilia: A disorder of the blood clotting system resulting in a tendency to form blood clots. It may also lead to a higher risk of miscarriage.

Thyroid-stimulating hormone (TSH): A hormone produced by the pituitary gland that stimulates the production of thyroid hormone from the thyroid gland.

Transvaginal ultrasound: An imaging technique that uses sound waves produced by a wand-like probe placed within the vagina.

Trisomy: An abnormal genetic condition that arises when an individual possesses three copies of a particular chromosome instead of the normal two copies.

Tubal ligation: Surgical sterilization of a woman, performed by cutting or occluding the fallopian tubes.

Tubal reanastamosis: A surgical procedure to repair the fallopian tubes following a tubal sterilization procedure.

U

Ultrasonography: A noninvasive imaging technology that uses sound waves to create images of various structures in the body.

Ureaplasma: A type of bacteria that may contribute to infertility.

Uterus: The pear-shaped organ that contains a growing pregnancy; in lay terms, "the womb."

V

Varicocele: One or more dilated veins often located in the scrotal sac and thought to be a possible cause of male infertility.

Varicocelectomy: Ligation of dilated testicular or inguinal veins thought to be a source of male infertility.

Vasectomy: Surgical sterilization of a man by cutting the vas deferens.

W

Wyden law: Legislation passed by the U.S. Congress and sponsored by Congressman Ron Wyden that regulates the advertising and reporting of IVF success rates by fertility clinics.

X

X-linked recessive disease: A genetic disease associated with a mutation on the X chromosome. A male carrying such a mutation will have the disorder because he has only one X chromosome, but a female carrying a mutation on just one X chromosome has a normal gene on the other chromosome and so will not be affected by the disease.

Z

Zona pellucida: The outer cellular membrane that surrounds the egg and embryo up to the blastocyst stage of development.

Index

Note: *Italic* page numbers indicate figures and tables.